# Thyroid Cancer: A Clinical Overview and A Useful Laboratory Manual

## Edited By

## Silvia Cantara

*Section of Endocrinology & Metabolism*
*Department of Internal Medicine*
*Endocrinology & Metabolism and Biochemistry*
*University of Siena*
*Siena*
*Italy*

# DEDICATION

*To my son Samuele, who makes me happy, proud and grateful every day*

# CONTENTS

# FOREWORD

*Thyroid Cancer: A Clinical Overview and a Useful Laboratory Manual* is a comprehensive eBook dealing with all aspects of thyroid cancer including the biology and the pathogenesis of thyroid nodule. *Silvia Cantara, the editor*, has integrated in this eBook, different aspects to consider different facets of thyroid cancer. There are chapters dealing with relevant basic science including the oncogenes involved in thyroid cancer development and the new markers useful in the diagnosis of thyroid cancer.

Thyroid nodules are frequent in the general population, especially in those countries with iodine deficiency. Thyroid tumors have a relatively high incidence. Thyroid tumors are an ideal model for the study of tumorigenesis in epithelial tissues.

Each chapter covers its topic in a didactic and understandable manner, also for the reader without expertise in that field.

Each chapter includes an up-to-date review of the literature, and in all chapters there are extensive citations. This eBook, not only underlined the aspect of the diagnostic procedures for thyroid nodule, but also the relevant role of oncogenes in the diagnosis and treatment, including the target therapy by tyrosine kinase inhibitors.

This eBook can be used as a practical, clinically-oriented text and as a reference. It will be of interest to use to a wide variety of physicians that treat and see patients with thyroid nodules and thyroid cancer.

*Dario Giuffrida*

Chief, Division of Oncology

Mediterranean Institute of Oncology

Viagrande, CT

Professor of Clinical Oncology

University of Catania

Italy

# PREFACE

Thyroid nodules are very frequent in the general population especially in those countries with iodide deficiency. The majority of thyroid nodules are benign and approximately 5% of thyroid nodules are cancer. In this view, it is very important the pre-surgical diagnosis to distinguish benign from malignant lesions in order to limit surgical treatment only to the malignant/suspicious nodules. Nowadays, fine needle aspiration cytology (FNAC) is the "gold standard" for the differential diagnosis of thyroid nodules. In general, in expert hands, it is associated with good specificity and acceptable sensitivity. However, this procedure has some limitations related to inadequate sampling or to the difficulty to discriminate follicular lesions. Therefore, a significant proportion of patients who do not have malignant lesions are submitted to unnecessary thyroidectomy. The discovery of genetic alterations specific for differentiated thyroid cancer may provide molecular markers to be searched for in the material obtained by FNA, thus increasing the diagnostic accuracy of traditional cytology.

Overall, this eBook describes the problems of FNAC limitations; previous experience on oncogenes search; laboratory limitations; new molecular techniques to refine diagnosis and the prognostic significance of each genetic alteration providing a critical and useful manual (together with a laboratory handbook) essential for students, young endocrinologist, family doctors but also for biologists and technicians involved in the pre-surgical diagnosis of thyroid cancer.

In chapter 1, the author has introduces the matter of thyroid nodules, their incidence in the general population, the percentage of malignant thyroid nodules and the benign lesions. Chapters 2-3 are dedicated to the methods for the diagnosis of thyroid nodules. Professor Pacini (author of chapter 2) is an internationally recognized authority in the field of thyroid cancer and thyroide diseases in general. His research has contributed to the diagnosis and treatment of thyroid cancer and he has been deeply involved in the study of the thyroid effects of the post-Cherbobyl radioactive fall-out. He contributed to this eBook with a well designed review on FNAC.

In chapters 4-5 oncogenes involved in thyroid tumorigenesis and methods for the routinary molecular analysis of these oncogenes in a thyroid aspirate, are described. The author is a post-doctoral researcher which contributed with Professor Pacini to one of the major internationally recognised paper on this subject.

Chapters 6-8 are dedicated to the problem of familial thyroid cancer, medullary thyroid cancer and the new approaches of the target theraphy for refractory cancers.

In the last chapter, possible new markers to be introduced in the diagnosis of thyroid cancer (*i.e.* telomerase, miRNA) are described with particular accent on their importance, specificity for thyroid cancer and problems related to their evaluation (*i.e.* can they be measured in blood or FNAC?; is their measurement easy to perform or time consuming?).

We would like to thank Bentham Science Publishers for their support and efforts.

*Silvia Cantara*

Section of Endocrinology & Metabolism
Department of Internal Medicine
Endocrinology & Metabolism and Biochemistry
University of Siena
Siena
Italy

# List of Contributors

**Furio Pacini**

Section of Endocrinology & Metabolism, Department of Internal Medicine, Endocrinology & Metabolism and Biochemistry, University of Siena, Siena, Italy

**Silvia Cantara**

Section of Endocrinology & Metabolism, Department of Internal Medicine, Endocrinology & Metabolism and Biochemistry, University of Siena, Siena, Italy

**Maria G. Castagna**

Section of Endocrinology & Metabolism, Department of Internal Medicine, Endocrinology & Metabolism and Biochemistry, University of Siena, Siena, Italy

**Paolo E. Macchia**

Department of Endocrinology, Molecular Oncology and Clinic University of Napoles "Federico II", Naples, Italy

**Stefania Marchisotta**

Section of Endocrinology & Metabolism, Department of Internal Medicine, Endocrinology & Metabolism and Biochemistry, University of Siena, Siena, Italy

**Tala J. H. Pablo**

Clinica Alemana, Vitacura 5951, Las Condes, Santiago, Chile

# ACKNOWLEDGEMENTS

I would like to thank Stefano Giardi for his help with PyMOL (v1.5) programme for the elaboration of DNA structure for cover image and Prof. Alexander Sorisky for his help with English language revision.

# CHAPTER 1

## Thyroid Nodules

### Furio Pacini[1] and Tala J. H. Pablo[2,*]

*[1]Section of Endocrinology & Metabolism, Department of Medical, Surgical and Neurological Sciences University of Siena, Siena, Italy and [2]Clinica Alemana, Vitacura 5951, Las Condes, Santiago, Chile*

**Abstract:** Thyroid nodules are frequently found in the overall population. The clinical relevance of evaluating thyroid nodules is to rule out thyroid cancer. After history, physical examination, and TSH determination, neck ultrasonography is the most important tool to evaluate the risk of a particular nodule to be cancer, and to select patients for FNA. This chapter discusses these aspects.

**Keywords:** Thyroid nodules, thyroid cancer, evaluation methods.

## INTRODUCTION AND EPIDEMIOLOGY

Thyroid nodules have been defined as "lesions within the thyroid gland, radiologically distinct from the surrounding thyroid parenchyma" [1], and are the manifestation of a wide range of conditions or diseases. Their prevalence by palpation on physical examination is reported to be between 4% and 7% [2, 3], whereas the prevalence of nodules detected by ultrasonography ranges between 20-76% of the adult population [3-6]. Thyroid nodules are most common in women and their prevalence increases in older patients especially in countries affected by moderate/severe iodine deficiency.

The major causes of thyroid nodules are listed in Table **1**. The most important aim

---

*Address correspondence to Tala J. H. Pablo: Clinica Alemana. Vitacura 5951, Las Condes, Santiago, Chile; Tel: +5622101328; Fax: +56977589245; E-mail: h_tala@hotmail.com

in the evaluation of thyroid nodules is to rule out thyroid cancer, which can occur in ~ 4% - 6.5% of all thyroid nodules [7-10]. Of these thyroid cancers, the most frequent is papillary thyroid carcinoma (80%-90%), followed by follicular thyroid cancer (10-20%). Much less frequent are medullary thyroid carcinoma (5-8%) and anaplastic thyroid carcinoma (<5%). Primary thyroid lymphoma and metastatic carcinoma to the thyroid are rare.

**Table 1:** Major causes of thyroid nodules

| ETIOLOGY OF THYROID NODULES | |
|---|---|
| **Benign Thyroid nodules** | **Malignant** |
| Cyst: Colloid, simple or hemorrhagic | Papillary thyroid carcinoma |
| Hashimoto`s thyroiditis | Follicular thyroid carcinoma |
| Follicular Adenoma/ Hürthle cell adenoma | Medullary thyroid carcinoma |
| Multinodular goiter | Anaplastic Thyroid Carcinoma |
| Subacute thyroiditis | Primary thyroid lymphoma |
| Thyroid Hemiagenesis | Metastatic carcinoma to the thyroid. |
| **Benign non Thyroid nodules** | |
| Thyroglossal cyst | |
| Parathyroid cyst or adenoma | |

## EVALUATION OF THYROID NODULES

In the past, thyroid nodules came to clinical attention mainly when noticed by the patient or as an incidental finding during physical examination. Nowadays, consultation for thyroid nodules are because they have been incidentally found during radiologic procedures such as carotid ultrasonography, computed tomography (CT) or positron emission tomography (PET) scanning. The prevalence of thyroid cancer in palpable nodules is the same as for nodules incidentally found by radiologic methods [11] but those found on PET scan are more frequently associated to thyroid cancer [12].

The evaluation of thyroid nodules includes history, physical examination, TSH measurement and thyroid ultrasonography in all patients. In Europe, serum calcitonin measurement is performed in all patients, but in the US this is not generally done. Thyroid scintigraphy, which was the most frequently radiologic tool used in the past, is of limited value and is indicated only when a functioning nodule is suspected (when TSH is low). After this initial evaluation, fine needle aspiration cytology (FNA) is performed in selected patients to better discriminate patients who may need surgery.

**History and Physical Examination**

The evaluation of thyroid nodules starts with the patient's history and physical examination. Clinical factors important to be considered are age, sex, family history of thyroid cancer and previous history of radiation to the neck.

The rate of malignancy of thyroid nodules is higher in patients younger than 30 years and older than 60 years compared to patients aged 30 to 60 years [9, 13]. Male sex has also been associated with a higher risk of cancer. Family history of thyroid cancer should always be considered. History of papillary thyroid carcinoma in a parent or sibling increases the risk of thyroid cancer by threefold and by six fold, respectively [14]. Family history of medullary thyroid carcinoma, pheochromocytoma, or hyperparathyroidism should increase suspicion for familial medullary thyroid carcinoma or MEN2 syndrome. Other rare familial syndromes should raise the suspicion for follicular cell derived thyroid carcinoma, such as Familial polyposis, Cowden Syndrome and Carney complex.

Previous exposure to head and neck radiotherapy [15, 16] and whole body radiation related to haematopoietic stem cell transplantation also increase the risk of thyroid cancer [17].

Recent development of the thyroid nodule, rapid growth, hoarseness and dysphagia should raise the suspicion of malignancy. Sudden swelling and tenderness may probably be secondary to a haemorrhage into a benign lesion. Tenderness, fever, and hyperthyroid symptoms should raise the suspicion of subacute thyroiditis. A nodule of stable size over years is probably benign, but does not rule out thyroid cancer.

On physical examination, enlarged lymph nodes or a very hard nodule fixed to the strap muscles or the trachea are alarming signs.

Even though history and physical examination are a relevant step in the evaluation of thyroid nodules, in most patients they give little information on the risk of a particular nodule to be cancerous. Therefore, additional tests are essential for the correct risk assessment of the nodule. TSH and neck ultrasonography are performed in every patient under evaluation for thyroid nodule. Depending on their results, other tests may be performed. Some, but not all, authors recommend the measurement of serum calcitonin in every patient with thyroid nodules.

## TSH

TSH levels should be measured in every patient evaluated for thyroid nodules but its levels are not helpful in the differential diagnosis of benign and malignant nodules. When TSH levels are low, the thyroid nodule may be hyper functioning and therefore thyroid scintigraphy should be performed. On the other hand, it has been observed that there is a direct correlation between the TSH levels and the risk of malignancy (higher risk of malignancy at higher TSH levels) [18] and also with the grade of aggressiveness [19-20], even when TSH is within the normal range.

## Calcitonin

Several studies have suggested that measurement of serum calcitonin in every patient with thyroid nodules may allow the diagnosis of medullary thyroid carcinoma at an earlier stage, improving the overall survival of this disease [21-24]. The use of pentagastrin improves the specificity of this test in patients with mildly elevated calcitonin levels. Most European authors recommend this evaluation in every patient with thyroid nodules. However, since pentagastrin is no longer available in the United States, the American Thyroid Association guidelines state that it is not possible to recommend in favour or against measurement of serum calcitonin in the evaluation of thyroid nodules [1].

## Thyroid Ultrasonography

Thyroid ultrasonography is the most important tool used in the detection and evaluation of thyroid nodule and should be performed in every patient. It provides relevant information on nodule dimensions, structure and characteristics that better estimate the risk of malignancy. It is clearly superior to thyroid scintigraphy [25], neck computer tomography or other radiologic tools [26]. It also allows the detection of other nodules not previously found on the physical examination and also allows for the observation of changes in size of the nodules over time. Its high sensitivity detects tiny lesions as small as 2-3 mm. Several features on the neck ultrasonography have been correlated with a higher risk of malignancy: hypoechogenicity, irregular or microlobulated margins, increased intranodular vascularity, microcalcifications and taller-than-wide shape, incomplete halo, and documented enlargement of a nodule over time [11, 27-31]. None of these features are sufficient to differentiate benign from malignant tumours, but a combination of 2 or more of them identify lesions that have a higher risk of malignancy. There are 2 ultrasonographic features that strongly predict the risk of malignancy: extracaspular invasion into peri-thyroid muscles and the presence of pathologic lymph nodes (*e.g.* microcalcifications and cystic changes). On the other hand, ultrasonographic features associated with a low risk of malignancy are: hyperechoic nodule, spongiform appearance and comet-tail shadowing [28]. The size of the nodule is not predictive of malignancy [11, 32].

## Elastography

This is a new dynamic ultrasonographic technique that assesses the hardness of the tissue as an indicator of malignancy. The use of this technique has been associated with a specificity of 96-100% and sensitivity of 82-97% in the diagnostic evaluation of thyroid nodules [33, 34]. It has also been found to be associated with a better classification of the risk of malignancy of nodules for which FNA results were indeterminate/follicular lesions [35]. Therefore, it seems to be a promising tool for the evaluation of thyroid nodules, but larger prospective studies are needed to establish the accuracy and clinical utility of this technique.

## Scintigraphy

The only indication to perform thyroid scintigraphy is when TSH levels are low. If thyroid scintigraphy shows a hyperfuncioning thyroid nodule, the risk of cancer is very low [36, 37] and cytological examination is not indicated, unless highly suspicious features on the neck ultrasound are found. Depending on the clinical scenario, hyperfunctioning tumours can be observed, or treated with radioactive iodine, antithyroid drugs or surgery.

## Fine Needle Aspiration (FNA) Biopsy for Cytologic Examination

FNA biopsy is the most accurate and reliable tool for diagnosing thyroid malignancy and selecting candidates for surgery [38, 39]. It is preferably performed under ultrasonography guidance in order to reduce the rates of false negative and non-diagnostic cytology. FNAB has an overall accuracy of 95%. The sensitivity is between 43-98% and the specificity is between 72-100%, with positive and negative predictive values of 89-98% and 94-99%, respectively [40]. False positive and false negative results are between 1-11% and 0-7%, respectively.

The decision of who should be referred for FNA depends on the patient's risk factors and the sonographic appearance of the nodule [41]. Risk factors include: history of thyroid cancer in one or more first-degree relatives; exposure to external beam radiation as a child; exposure to ionizing radiation in childhood or adolescence; prior hemithyroidectomy with discovery of thyroid cancer; FDG avidity on PET scanning; MEN2/FMTC associated RET proto-oncogenic mutation and calcitonin > 100 pg/mL. Suspicious features on ultrasound include: microcalcifications, hypoechoic appearance; increased nodular vascularity; infiltrative margins and taller than wide dimensions on transverse view [1]. Using theses features, the current ATA guidelines for the management of thyroid nodules recommend performing FNA cytological examination in the following cases: 1) when suspicious lymph nodes are present (regardless of nodule size) (recommendation A); 2) hypoechoic nodules or when microcalcifications are present and the nodules size is ≥ 1 cm (recommendation B); 3) in nodules that are iso or hyperechoic, FNA is recommended when size is ≥ 1-1.5 cm (recommendation C); 4) in mixed cystic-solid nodules, FNA is recommended when any suspicious features are found and nodule is ≥ 1.5-2.0 cm (recommendation B) and when nodule is ≥ 2.0 cm if no suspicious feature is found (recommendation C). In case of spongiform nodules, the risk of cancer is extremely low, and therefore recommendations are to perform FNA only in nodules ≥ 2.0 cm, although observation alone is an option (recommendation C). In purely cystic nodules, FNA is not recommended. When a high-risk history is present, the authors recommend FNA for all patients with nodules ≥ 5 mm when suspicious sonographic features are present (recommendation A), but they were not able to recommend for or against FNA in nodules ≥ 5 mm when no suspicious sonographic features were present (recommendation I) ]. It is a matter of debate how to proceed in the evaluation of nodules < 1.0 cm in patients with no risk factors. The ATA guidelines do not recommend FNA in nodules < 1.0 cm with no high-risk history, regardless of ultrasound features. However, many authors suggest FNA for nodules <1.0 cm with suspicious features on neck ultrasound.

Recently, a group developed a classification for the cancer risk of a thyroid nodule, similar to the BIRADS classification for breast cancer. This is the TIRADS classification [40], in which nodules were classified with scores 1 to 5.

The risk of thyroid cancer in this study was 0% for TIRADS 2, 3.4% for TIRADS 3, 14% for TIRADS 4, and 86.5% for TIRADS 5 (what happened to TIRADS 1?).

When the FNA results clearly indicate a benign nodule, observation is indicated, unless there are local symptoms from a very large nodule or the nodule is hyperfunctioning.

## CONCLUSIONS

Thyroid nodules are frequently found in the overall population. The clinical relevance of the evaluation for thyroid nodules is to rule out the presence of thyroid cancer. After history, physical examination, and TSH determination, neck ultrasonography is the most important tool for evaluating the cancer risk of specific nodules, and for selecting patients for FNA. As a general rule, all mixed or solid nodules should be submitted to FNAB. When a goiter is multinodular, FNAB should be done in those which are hypofunctioning on scintigraphy and have the most suspicious findings on thyroid US. In cystic nodules, FNAB is mainly carried out with a therapeutic intent (evacuation) but also as a diagnostic procedure to identify the very rare cystic carcinoma. When FNA results are clearly indicative of a benign nodule, observation is recommended, unless symptoms related to a large or hyperfunctioning nodule are present.

## CONFLICT OF INTEREST

The authors confirm that they have no conflicts of interest.

## ACKNOWLEDGEMENTS

None Declared.

# REFERENCES

[1]     Cooper, D.S., Doherty, G.M., Haugen, B.R., Kloos, R.T., Lee, S.L., Mandel, S.J., Mazzaferri, E.L., McIver, B., Pacini, F., Schlumberger, M., *et al.* Revised American Thyroid Association management guidelines for patients with thyroid nodules and differentiated thyroid cancer. Thyroid 2009, 19:1167-1214.

[2]     Singer, P.A., Cooper, D.S., Daniels, G.H., Ladenson, P.W., Greenspan, F.S., Levy, E.G.,Braverman, L.E., Clark, O.H., McDougall, I.R., Ain, K.V., *et al.* Treatment guidelines for patients with thyroid nodules and well-differentiated thyroid cancer. American Thyroid Association. Arch Intern Med 1996, 156:2165-2172.

[3]     Mazzaferri, E.L. Management of a solitary thyroid nodule. N Engl J Med 1993, 328:553-559.

[4]     Ezzat, S., Sarti, D.A., Cain, D.R., and Braunstein, G.D. 1994. Thyroid incidentalomas. Prevalence by palpation and ultrasonography. *Arch Intern Med* 154:1838-1840.

[5]     Tan, G.H., and Gharib, H. Thyroid incidentalomas: management approaches to nonpalpable nodules discovered incidentally on thyroid imaging. Ann Intern Med 1997, 126:226-231.

[6]     Guth, S., Theune, U., Aberle, J., Galach, A., and Bamberger, C.M. Very high prevalence of thyroid nodules detected by high frequency (13 MHz) ultrasound examination. Eur J Clin Invest 2009, 39:699-706.

[7]     Hegedus, L. Clinical practice. The thyroid nodule. N Engl J Med 2004, 351:1764-1771.

[8]     Werk, E.E., Jr., Vernon, B.M., Gonzalez, J.J., Ungaro, P.C., and McCoy, R.C. Cancer in thyroid nodules. A community hospital survey. Arch Intern Med 1994, 144:474-476.

[9]     Belfiore, A., Giuffrida, D., La Rosa, G.L., Ippolito, O., Russo, G., Fiumara, A., Vigneri, R., and Filetti, S. High frequency of cancer in cold thyroid nodules occurring at young age. Acta Endocrinol (Copenh) 1989, 121:197-202.

[10]    Lin, J.D., Chao, T.C., Huang, B.Y., Chen, S.T., Chang, H.Y., and Hsueh, C. Thyroid cancer in the thyroid nodules evaluated by ultrasonography and fine-needle aspiration cytology. Thyroid 2005, 15:708-717.

[11]    Papini, E., Guglielmi, R., Bianchini, A., Crescenzi, A., Taccogna, S., Nardi, F., Panunzi, C., Rinaldi, R., Toscano, V., and Pacella, C.M. Risk of malignancy in nonpalpable thyroid nodules: predictive value of ultrasound and color-Doppler features. J Clin Endocrinol Metab 2002, 87:1941-1946.

[12]    Soelberg, K.K., Bonnema, S.J., Brix, T., and Hegedus, L. Risk of malignancy in thyroid incidentalomas detected by 18F-fluorodeoxyglucose positron emission tomography. A systematic review. Thyroid 2012

[13]    Belfiore, A., La Rosa, G.L., La Porta, G.A., Giuffrida, D., Milazzo, G., Lupo, L., Regalbuto, C., and Vigneri, R. 1992. Cancer risk in patients with cold thyroid nodules: relevance of iodine intake, sex, age, and multinodularity. Am J Med 1992, 93:363-369.

[14]   Hemminki, K., Eng, C., and Chen, B. Familial risks for nonmedullary thyroid cancer. J Clin Endocrinol Metab 2005, 90:5747-5753.

[15]   Favus, M.J., Schneider, A.B., Stachura, M.E., Arnold, J.E., Ryo, U.Y., Pinsky, S.M., Colman, M., Arnold, M.J., and Frohman, L.A. Thyroid cancer occurring as a late consequence of head-and-neck irradiation. Evaluation of 1056 patients. N Engl J Med 1976, 294:1019-1025.

[16]   Cerletty, J.M., Guansing, A.R., Engbring, N.H., Hagen, T.C., Kim, H.J., Shetty, K.R., Rosenfeld, P.S., and Wilson, S. Radiation-related thyroid carcinoma. Arch Surg 1978, 113:1072-1076.

[17]   Cohen, A., Rovelli, A., Merlo, D.F., van Lint, M.T., Lanino, E., Bresters, D., Ceppi, M., Bocchini, V., Tichelli, A., and Socie, G. Risk for secondary thyroid carcinoma after hematopoietic stem-cell transplantation: an EBMT Late Effects Working Party Study. J Clin Oncol 2007, 25:2449-2454.

[18]   Boelaert, K., Horacek, J., Holder, R.L., Watkinson, J.C., Sheppard, M.C., and Franklyn, J.A. Serum thyrotropin concentration as a novel predictor of malignancy in thyroid nodules investigated by fine-needle aspiration. J Clin Endocrinol Metab 2006, 91:4295-4301.

[19]   Haymart, M.R., Repplinger, D.J., Leverson, G.E., Elson, D.F., Sippel, R.S., Jaume, J.C., and Chen, H. Higher serum thyroid stimulating hormone level in thyroid nodule patients is associated with greater risks of differentiated thyroid cancer and advanced tumor stage. J Clin Endocrinol Metab 2008, 93:809-814.

[20]   Pacini, F., Pinchera, A., Giani, C., Grasso, L., Doveri, F., and Baschieri, L. Serum thyroglobulin in thyroid carcinoma and other thyroid disorders. J Endocrinol Invest 1980, 3:283-292.

[21]   Elisei, R., Bottici, V., Luchetti, F., Di Coscio, G., Romei, C., Grasso, L., Miccoli, P., Iacconi, P., Basolo, F., Pinchera, A., *et al.* Impact of routine measurement of serum calcitonin on the diagnosis and outcome of medullary thyroid cancer: experience in 10,864 patients with nodular thyroid disorders. J Clin Endocrinol Metab 2004, 89:163-168.

[22]   Hahm, J.R., Lee, M.S., Min, Y.K., Lee, M.K., Kim, K.W., Nam, S.J., Yang, J.H., and Chung, J.H. Routine measurement of serum calcitonin is useful for early detection of medullary thyroid carcinoma in patients with nodular thyroid diseases. Thyroid 2001, 11:73-80.

[23]   Niccoli, P., Wion-Barbot, N., Caron, P., Henry, J.F., de Micco, C., Saint Andre, J.P., Bigorgne, J.C., Modigliani, E., and Conte-Devolx, B. Interest of routine measurement of serum calcitonin: study in a large series of thyroidectomized patients. The French Medullary Study Group. J Clin Endocrinol Metab 1997, 82:338-341.

[24]   Costante, G., Meringolo, D., Durante, C., Bianchi, D., Nocera, M., Tumino, S., Crocetti, U., Attard, M., Maranghi, M., Torlontano, M., *et al.* Predictive value of serum calcitonin levels for preoperative diagnosis of medullary thyroid carcinoma in a cohort of 5817 consecutive patients with thyroid nodules. J Clin Endocrinol Metab 2007, 92:450-455.

[25]  Solbiati, L., Volterrani, L., Rizzatto, G., Bazzocchi, M., Busilacci, P., Candiani, F., Ferrari, F., Giuseppetti, G., Maresca, G., Mirk, P., *et al.* The thyroid gland with low uptake lesions: evaluation by ultrasound. Radiology 1985, 155:187-191.

[26]  Radecki, P.D., Arger, P.H., Arenson, R.L., Jennings, A.S., Coleman, B.G., Mintz, M.C., and Kressel, H.Y. Thyroid imaging: comparison of high-resolution real-time ultrasound and computed tomography. Radiology 1984, 153:145-147.

[27]  Hong, Y.J., Son, E.J., Kim, E.K., Kwak, J.Y., Hong, S.W., and Chang, H.S. 2010. Positive predictive values of sonographic features of solid thyroid nodule. Clin Imaging 2010, 34:127-133.

[28]   Moon, W.J., Jung, S.L., Lee, J.H., Na, D.G., Baek, J.H., Lee, Y.H., Kim, J., Kim, H.S., Byun, J.S., and Lee, D.H. Benign and malignant thyroid nodules: US differentiation--multicenter retrospective study. Radiology 2008, 247:762-770.

[29]  Frates, M.C., Benson, C.B., Charboneau, J.W., Cibas, E.S., Clark, O.H., Coleman, B.G., Cronan, J.J., Doubilet, P.M., Evans, D.B., Goellner, J.R., *et al.* Management of thyroid nodules detected at US: Society of Radiologists in Ultrasound consensus conference statement. Radiology 2005, 237:794-800.

[30]  Rago, T., Vitti, P., Chiovato, L., Mazzeo, S., De Liperi, A., Miccoli, P., Viacava, P., Bogazzi, F., Martino, E., and Pinchera, A. Role of conventional ultrasonography and color flow-doppler sonography in predicting malignancy in 'cold' thyroid nodules. Eur J Endocrinol 1998, 138:41-46.

[31]  Mandel, S.J. Diagnostic use of ultrasonography in patients with nodular thyroid disease. Endocr Pract 2004, 0:246-252.

[32]  Kim, E.K., Park, C.S., Chung, W.Y., Oh, K.K., Kim, D.I., Lee, J.T., and Yoo, H.S. New sonographic criteria for recommending fine-needle aspiration biopsy of nonpalpable solid nodules of the thyroid. AJR Am J Roentgenol 2002, 178:687-691.

[33]  Rago, T., Santini, F., Scutari, M., Pinchera, A., and Vitti, P. Elastography: new developments in ultrasound for predicting malignancy in thyroid nodules. J Clin Endocrinol Metab 2007, 92:2917-2922.

[34]  Bojunga, J., Herrmann, E., Meyer, G., Weber, S., Zeuzem, S., and Friedrich-Rust, M. Real-time elastography for the differentiation of benign and malignant thyroid nodules: a meta-analysis. Thyroid 2010, 20:1145-1150.

[35]  Rago, T., Scutari, M., Santini, F., Loiacono, V., Piaggi, P., Di Coscio, G., Basolo, F., Berti, P., Pinchera, A., and Vitti, P. Real-time elastosonography: useful tool for refining the presurgical diagnosis in thyroid nodules with indeterminate or nondiagnostic cytology. J Clin Endocrinol Metab 2010, 95:5274-5280.

[36]  Fiore, E., Rago, T., Provenzale, M.A., Scutari, M., Ugolini, C., Basolo, F., Di Coscio, G., Berti, P., Grasso, L., Elisei, R., *et al.* Lower levels of TSH are associated with a lower risk of papillary thyroid cancer in patients with thyroid nodular disease: thyroid autonomy may play a protective role. Endocr Relat Cancer 2009, 16:1251-1260.

[37]     Meller, J., and Becker, W. 2002. The continuing importance of thyroid scintigraphy in the era of high-resolution ultrasound. Eur J Nucl Med Mol Imaging 2009, 29:S425-438.

[38]     Castro, M.R., and Gharib, H. Thyroid fine-needle aspiration biopsy: progress, practice, and pitfalls. Endocr Pract 2003, 9:128-136.

[39]     Gharib, H., and Goellner, J.R. Fine-needle aspiration biopsy of the thyroid: an appraisal. Ann Intern Med 1993, 118:282-289.

[40]     Gharib H, Goellner JR, Johnson DA. Fine needle aspiration of the thyroid. A 12 year experience with 11,000 biopsies. Clin Lab Med 1993, 13:699-709.

[41]     Horvath, E., Majlis, S., Rossi, R., Franco, C., Niedmann, J.P., Castro, A., and Dominguez, M. An ultrasonogram reporting system for thyroid nodules stratifying cancer risk for clinical management. J Clin Endocrinol Metab 2009, 94:1748-1751.

*Send Orders for Reprints on reprints@benthamscience.net*

# CHAPTER 2

## Alternative Methods for the Diagnosis of Thyroid Nodules

**Paolo E. Macchia**[*]

*Department of Endocrinology, Molecular Oncology and Clinic University of Napoles "Federico II", Naples, Italy*

**Abstract:** Thyroid nodules can be identified in approximately 5% of the population. The American Thyroid Association guidelines indicate fine needle aspiration as the most accurate method for the evaluation of a thyroid nodule; however in up to 20% of cases, cytology produces indeterminate or suspicious results that require surgery to complete the diagnosis. This chapter reviews molecular markers, which can be detected using protein-based assays, to improve the sensitivity of FNA.

**Keywords**: Galectin-3, HBME-1, CK-19, CD44v6, HMGI(Y), TPO.

## INTRODUCTION

Fine-needle aspiration biopsy (FNA) is considered to be the most cost-effective diagnostic test available for evaluation of thyroid nodules, and one of the primary goals of fine-needle aspiration biopsy is to avoid unnecessary surgery.

Benign nodules are identified in 60–70% of patients after FNA and malignant nodules occur in approximately 5% of cases. However, 10-30% of FNAs of thyroid nodules yield indeterminate or suspicious results, and surgical treatment is required for further evaluations. Fortunately, only 20–25% of these nodules are malignant, but with the consequence that that the large majority of patients (75–

*****Address correspondence to Paolo E. Macchia:** Department of Endocrinology, Molecular Oncology and Clinic University of Napoles "Federico II", Naples, Italy; Email: paoloemidio.macchia@unina.it

80%) undergo unnecessary surgical procedures. On the basis of these data, the revised guidelines of the American Thyroid Association have provided a level C recommendation in support of the use of molecular markers in patients with indeterminate cytology on FNA [1].

A useful molecular marker for cytological diagnosis must be able to reliably distinguish between malignant or benign lesions (mostly in indeterminate nodules) and must be easily measured from products of FNAs either by immunocytochemistry methods or by RT-PCR.

In this chapter, genetic markers will not be presented. We will focus on the immunohistochemistry (IHC) assays, that, contrary to PCR-based methods, can be performed in most clinical laboratories [2].

## GALECTIN-3

Galectins are carbohydrate-binding proteins that are members of the β-galactoside binding lectin family. Galectins are expressed in epithelial and immune cells, and are involved in several cellular functions including cell growth, cycle regulation, tumorigenesis, and apoptosis [3].

*In vitro*, Galectin-3 (Gal-3) has been demonstrated to be necessary for the maintenance of transformed thyroid papillary cancer cell lines [4]. Gal-3 is one of the most studied markers in thyroid malignancy. Its usage in the detection of thyroid malignancy in indeterminate or suspicious FNA has a sensitivity that ranges from 20% to 100% and a specificity from 62% to 100% [5-10]. The Italian Thyroid Cancer Study performed one of the largest prospective multicenter study on the role of Gal-3 as molecular maker in patients with indeterminate cytology on FNA. The study included 544 patients and immunohistochemistry for Gal-3 revealed a sensitivity of 78% and specificity of 93% [11].

In summary, galectin-3 protein is one of the more clinically useful markers for the diagnosis of thyroid nodules. It is highly expressed in malignant but not in normal thyroid tissue, the assay can be easily performed on both surgical and FNA samples and Gal-3 antibodies for immunohistochemistry are commercially available. In the case of an in determinate FNA with positive staining for Gal-3, surgery is strongly recommended. However, no specific suggestions can be made in the case of Gal-3 negative staining [9].

By contrast, several authors do not believe that Gal-3 testing is useful to distinguish between benign and malignant lesions and have criticized this method [12-14]. This suggests that galectin-3 immunodetection is potentially useful only in the context of other markers.

## HBME-1

Hector Battiflora Mesothelial-1 (HBME-1) is a monoclonal antibody developed against the microvillous surface of mesothelial cells. HBME-1 plays an important role in the stimulation of cancer cell proliferation and migration. It has been used in differential diagnosis of mesothelioma and adenocarcinoma [15] and subsequently applied to the diagnosis of malignant thyroid conditions [16]. HBME-1 is highly expressed in both papillary (PTC) and follicular (FTC) thyroid carcinomas with little expression in medullary and anaplastic thyroid carcinomas. De Micco *et al.* noticed that HBME-1 is not expressed in benign thyroid lesion but expressed in malignant thyroid cancer, indicating HBME-1 is the most specific marker for thyroid malignancy and may be useful in differentiating malignant thyroid cancer from benign tumor, mostly PTC [17].

HBME-1 immunocytochemistry had a sensitivity of 79–87% and a specificity of 83–96% in FNA samples with indeterminate or suspicious cytology [7, 18]. HBME-1 may be useful as a suitable marker for the IHC due to its high sensitivity and specificity. However, its prognostic importance needs to be addressed. It is very likely that HBME-1 will be useful in combination with other markers as part of a panel [19].

## CK-19

Cytokeratin 19 (CK19) is the smallest of 20 members of the cytokeratin family that is part of the intra-cytoplasmic cytoskeleton of epithelial cells [20]. CK-19 expression was often found altered in different types of epithelial malignancies with high sensitivity but poor specificity, including endometrial cancer, bladder cancer and breast cancers [21]. CK-19 is also expressed in thyroid cancer. Positive CK-19 staining is present in FNA samples from PTC [22], but its expression is not particularly useful in follicular lesions [23]. The average sensitivity and specificity of CK-19 for differentiating benign from malignant thyroid tumor is 80.4% and 72% respectively [24]. Despite its low specificity, CK-19 can be useful in the diagnosis of thyroid cancers as part of a panel of other biomarkers.

## CD44V6

CD44 is a polymorphic family of immunologically related cell-surface glycoproteins, which have a functional role in regulating several physiological and pathophysiological processes, including cell-cell and cell-matrix interactions, cell migration, and tumor growth and progression [25, 26].

Chhieng and colleagues [27] reported that CD44v6 is useful in differentiating PTC from other thyroid lesions with nuclear grooves. Bartolazzi *et al.* [10] demonstrated that CD44v6 was positive in 72% to 100% of carcinomas, but in benign proliferative lesions was present in 38% to 100%. This finding discouraged the use of CD44v6 immunodetection for discriminating benign proliferative from malignant thyroid lesions. Despite such discouraging results, the same study of Bartolazzi showed that co-expression of CD44v6 and Galectin-

3 showed a very high sensitivity (88%), specificity (98%), positive predictive value (91%) and diagnostic accuracy (97%), suggesting that CD44v6 may strengthen the significance of Galectin-3 expression in well-differentiated follicular lesions [10].

## HMGI(Y)

The high mobility group I (Y) protein [HMGI(Y)] belongs to a group of nuclear proteins involved in modulation of chromatin structure and function. Chiappeta *et al.* found HMGI(Y) expression in 96% of malignant thyroid tumors, but in only 20% of benign lesions by immunohistochemistry, as well as only in 4 FNA samples of thyroid nodules that were diagnosed as carcinomas after surgery out of the 12 examined [28]. Subsequently, Czyz *et al.* [29] showed that HMGI(Y) gene expression was detected only in follicular carcinomas, whereas in papillary carcinomas, follicular adenomas, and control tissues, there was no evidence of HMGI(Y) expression. Thus, HMGI(Y) protein might serve as a marker for follicular carcinoma in FNA biopsy samples [30].

## TPO

Thyroid peroxidase (TPO) is a membrane thyroid enzyme essential for thyroid hormone synthesis. It is present in large quantity in the cytoplasm of all benign follicular thyroid cells. In malignant tumors, TPO synthesis is reduced to varying degrees [31, 32]: it is still present in differentiated thyroid carcinomas at the early stages, but its sensitivity and specificity in differentiating benign as it is expressed both in inflammatory and hyperplastic thyroid nodules [33].

The use of TPO in discriminating between benign and malignant lesions is still under debate. According to gene expression profiling analysis in thyroid cancer *versus* non-cancer, TPO was one of the top 12 candidate markers in terms of diagnostic utility [2]. A monoclonal antibody is commercially available [34], but other studies do not consider TPO very useful in the diagnosis of undefined thyroid nodules [24].

## PANELS OF SEVERAL MARKERS

The usage of different markers has been tested to improve the diagnostic efficacy in FNA, however so far none of the tested molecules has provided sufficient sensitivity and specificity evaluating specimens of indeterminate cytology.

The combination of immunohistochemistry panels provides only a marginal diagnostic advantage in comparison to the use of individual ones [2,35].

Several authors are still working to identify novel potential markers, and very recently, Troncone *et al.* published a retrospective study on 51 cases with FNA suspicious for Hurthle cell neoplasm. The authors used cyclins D1 and D3 as molecular markers, and achieved excellent sensitivity (100%) and specificity (94%) [36].

## CONCLUSIONS

Several national and international guidelines have helped to formalize the nomenclature associated with the indeterminate and suspicious thyroid nodules [1,37,38]. The use of molecular markers has been useful in several cases, however it needs to account for inter- and intra-observer differences in cytological diagnoses [39].

To assess their efficacy, additional studies that are multi-institutional and blinded to final histological results need to be performed on FNA samples that are indeterminate and suspicious. Finally, a great effort should be applied to demonstrate the clinical impact that one or more markers may have on patient management.

## CONFLICT OF INTEREST

The author confirms he has no conflicts of interest.

## ACKNOWLEDGEMENTS

Declared none.

## REFERENCES

[1]     Cooper DS, Doherty GM, Haugen BR, Kloos RT, Lee SL, Mandel SJ, *et al.* Revised American Thyroid Association management guidelines for patients with thyroid nodules and differentiated thyroid cancer. Thyroid: official journal of the American Thyroid Association. 2009 Nov;19(11):1167-214.

[2]     Griffith OL, Chiu CG, Gown AM, Jones SJ, Wiseman SM. Biomarker panel diagnosis of thyroid cancer: a critical review. Expert review of anticancer therapy. 2008 Sep;8(9):1399-413.

[3]     Liu FT, Rabinovich GA. Galectins as modulators of tumour progression. Nature reviews Cancer. 2005 Jan;5(1):29-41.

[4]     Yoshii T, Inohara H, Takenaka Y, Honjo Y, Akahani S, Nomura T, *et al.* Galectin-3 maintains the transformed phenotype of thyroid papillary carcinoma cells. International journal of oncology. 2001 Apr;18(4):787-92.

[5]     Sapio MR, Guerra A, Posca D, Limone PP, Deandrea M, Motta M, *et al.* Combined analysis of galectin-3 and BRAFV600E improves the accuracy of fine-needle aspiration biopsy with cytological findings suspicious for papillary thyroid carcinoma. Endocrine-related cancer. 2007 Dec;14(4):1089-97.

[6]     Bryson PC, Shores CG, Hart C, Thorne L, Patel MR, Richey L, *et al.* Immunohistochemical distinction of follicular thyroid adenomas and follicular carcinomas. Archives of otolaryngology--head & neck surgery. 2008 Jun;134(6):581-6.

[7]     Torregrossa L, Faviana P, Filice ME, Materazzi G, Miccoli P, Vitti P, *et al.* CXC chemokine receptor 4 immunodetection in the follicular variant of papillary thyroid carcinoma: comparison to galectin-3 and hector battifora mesothelial cell-1. Thyroid: official journal of the American Thyroid Association. 2010 May;20(5):495-504.

[8]     Saggiorato E, De Pompa R, Volante M, Cappia S, Arecco F, Dei Tos AP, *et al.* Characterization of thyroid 'follicular neoplasms' in fine-needle aspiration cytological specimens using a panel of immunohistochemical markers: a proposal for clinical application. Endocrine-related cancer. 2005 Jun;12(2):305-17.

[9]     Raggio E, Camandona M, Solerio D, Martino P, Franchello A, Orlandi F, *et al.* The diagnostic accuracy of the immunocytochemical markers in the pre-operative evaluation of follicular thyroid lesions. Journal of endocrinological investigation. 2010 Jun;33(6):378-81.

[10]  Bartolazzi A, Gasbarri A, Papotti M, Bussolati G, Lucante T, Khan A, *et al.* Application of an immunodiagnostic method for improving preoperative diagnosis of nodular thyroid lesions. Lancet. 2001 May 26;357(9269):1644-50.

[11]  Bartolazzi A, Orlandi F, Saggiorato E, Volante M, Arecco F, Rossetto R, *et al.* Galectin-3-expression analysis in the surgical selection of follicular thyroid nodules with indeterminate fine-needle aspiration cytology: a prospective multicentre study. The lancet oncology. 2008 Jun;9(6):543-9.

[12]  Bartolazzi A, Bussolati G. Galectin-3 does not reliably distinguish benign from malignant thyroid neoplasms. Histopathology. 2006 Jan;48(2):212-3.

[13]  Mehrotra P, Okpokam A, Bouhaidar R, Johnson SJ, Wilson JA, Davies BR, *et al.* Galectin-3 does not reliably distinguish benign from malignant thyroid neoplasms. Histopathology. 2004 Nov;45(5):493-500.

[14]  Sanabria A, Carvalho AL, Piana de Andrade V, Pablo Rodrigo J, Vartanian JG, Rinaldo A, *et al.* Is galectin-3 a good method for the detection of malignancy in patients with thyroid nodules and a cytologic diagnosis of "follicular neoplasm"? A critical appraisal of the evidence. Head & neck. 2007 Nov;29(11):1046-54.

[15]  Miettinen M, Karkkainen P. Differential reactivity of HBME-1 and CD15 antibodies in benign and malignant thyroid tumours. Preferential reactivity with malignant tumours. Virchows Archiv: an international journal of pathology. 1996 Nov;429(4-5):213-9.

[16]  Raphael SJ. The meanings of markers: ancillary techniques in diagnosis of thyroid neoplasia. Endocrine pathology. 2002 Winter;13(4):301-11.

[17]  de Micco C, Savchenko V, Giorgi R, Sebag F, Henry JF. Utility of malignancy markers in fine-needle aspiration cytology of thyroid nodules: comparison of Hector Battifora mesothelial antigen-1, thyroid peroxidase and dipeptidyl aminopeptidase IV. British journal of cancer. 2008 Feb 26;98(4):818-23.

[18]  Franco C, Martinez V, Allamand JP, Medina F, Glasinovic A, Osorio M, *et al.* Molecular markers in thyroid fine-needle aspiration biopsy: a prospective study. Applied immunohistochemistry & molecular morphology: AIMM / official publication of the Society for Applied Immunohistochemistry. 2009 May;17(3):211-5.

[19]  Kato MA, Fahey TJ, 3rd. Molecular markers in thyroid cancer diagnostics. The Surgical clinics of North America. 2009 Oct;89(5):1139-55.

[20]  Moll R, Divo M, Langbein L. The human keratins: biology and pathology. Histochemistry and cell biology. 2008 Jun;129(6):705-33.

[21]  Kwaspen FH, Smedts FM, Broos A, Bulten H, Debie WM, Ramaekers FC. Reproducible and highly sensitive detection of the broad spectrum epithelial marker keratin 19 in routine cancer diagnosis. Histopathology. 1997 Dec;31(6):503-16.

[22]  Khurana KK, Truong LD, LiVolsi VA, Baloch ZW. Cytokeratin 19 immunolocalization in cell block preparation of thyroid aspirates. An adjunct to fine-needle aspiration diagnosis of papillary thyroid carcinoma. Archives of pathology & laboratory medicine. 2003 May;127(5):579-83.

[23]     Beesley MF, McLaren KM. Cytokeratin 19 and galectin-3 immunohistochemistry in the differential diagnosis of solitary thyroid nodules. Histopathology. 2002 Sep;41(3):236-43.

[24]     Sethi K, Sarkar S, Das S, Mohanty B, Mandal M. Biomarkers for the diagnosis of thyroid cancer. Journal of experimental therapeutics & oncology. 2010;8(4):341-52.

[25]     Naor D, Sionov RV, Ish-Shalom D. CD44: structure, function, and association with the malignant process. Advances in cancer research. 1997;71:241-319.

[26]     Gunthert U, Hofmann M, Rudy W, Reber S, Zoller M, Haussmann I, *et al.* A new variant of glycoprotein CD44 confers metastatic potential to rat carcinoma cells. Cell. 1991 Apr 5;65(1):13-24.

[27]     Chhieng DC, Ross JS, McKenna BJ. CD44 immunostaining of thyroid fine-needle aspirates differentiates thyroid papillary carcinoma from other lesions with nuclear grooves and inclusions. Cancer. 1997 Jun 25;81(3):157-62.

[28]     Chiappetta G, Bandiera A, Berlingieri MT, Visconti R, Manfioletti G, Battista S, *et al.* The expression of the high mobility group HMGI (Y) proteins correlates with the malignant phenotype of human thyroid neoplasias. Oncogene. 1995 Apr 6;10(7):1307-14.

[29]     Czyz W, Balcerczak E, Jakubiak M, Pasieka Z, Kuzdak K, Mirowski M. HMGI(Y) gene expression as a potential marker of thyroid follicular carcinoma. Langenbeck's archives of surgery Deutsche Gesellschaft fur Chirurgie. 2004 Jun;389(3):193-7.

[30]     Rodrigo JP, Rinaldo A, Devaney KO, Shaha AR, Ferlito A. Molecular diagnostic methods in the diagnosis and follow-up of well-differentiated thyroid carcinoma. Head & neck. 2006 Nov;28(11):1032-9.

[31]     De Micco C, Kopp F, Vassko V, Grino M. *In situ* hybridization and immunohistochemistry study of thyroid peroxidase expression in thyroid tumors. Thyroid: official journal of the American Thyroid Association. 2000 Feb;10(2):109-15.

[32]     Di Cristofaro J, Silvy M, Lanteaume A, Marcy M, Carayon P, De Micco C. Expression of tpo mRNA in thyroid tumors: quantitative PCR analysis and correlation with alterations of ret, Braf, ras and pax8 genes. Endocrine-related cancer. 2006 Jun;13(2):485-95.

[33]     Schlumberger M, Lacroix L, Russo D, Filetti S, Bidart JM. Defects in iodide metabolism in thyroid cancer and implications for the follow-up and treatment of patients. Nature clinical practice Endocrinology & metabolism. 2007 Mar;3(3):260-9.

[34]     De Micco C, Ruf J, Chrestian MA, Gros N, Henry JF, Carayon P. Immunohistochemical study of thyroid peroxidase in normal, hyperplastic, and neoplastic human thyroid tissues. Cancer. 1991 Jun 15;67(12):3036-41.

[35]     Saleh HA, Feng J, Tabassum F, Al-Zohaili O, Husain M, Giorgadze T. Differential expression of galectin-3, CK19, HBME1, and Ret oncoprotein in the diagnosis of thyroid neoplasms by fine needle aspiration biopsy. CytoJournal. 2009;6:18.

[36]     Troncone G, Volante M, Iaccarino A, Zeppa P, Cozzolino I, Malapelle U, *et al.* Cyclin D1 and D3 overexpression predicts malignant behavior in thyroid fine-needle aspirates suspicious for Hurthle cell neoplasms. Cancer. 2009 Dec 25;117(6):522-9.

[37]  Baloch ZW, LiVolsi VA, Asa SL, Rosai J, Merino MJ, Randolph G, *et al.* Diagnostic terminology and morphologic criteria for cytologic diagnosis of thyroid lesions: a synopsis of the National Cancer Institute Thyroid Fine-Needle Aspiration State of the Science Conference. Diagnostic cytopathology. 2008 Jun;36(6):425-37.

[38]  Gharib H, Papini E, Paschke R, Duick DS, Valcavi R, Hegedus L, *et al.* American Association of Clinical Endocrinologists, Associazione Medici Endocrinologi, and European Thyroid Association medical guidelines for clinical practice for the diagnosis and management of thyroid nodules: Executive Summary of recommendations. Journal of endocrinological investigation. 2010 May;33(5):287-91.

[39]  Kouniavsky G, Zeiger MA. The quest for diagnostic molecular markers for thyroid nodules with indeterminate or suspicious cytology. Journal of surgical oncology. 2012 Apr 1;105(5):438-43.

# CHAPTER 3

# Oncogenes Involved in Thyroid Cancer Development

## Silvia Cantara[*]

*Section of Endocrinology & Metabolism, Department of Internal Medicine, Endocrinology & Metabolism and Biochemistry, University of Siena, Siena, Italy*

**Abstract:** Indeterminate nodules at FNAC are usually candidates for surgical therapy, but, at final histology, most of them are benign. An alternative to improve the diagnostic accuracy of FNAC might be the identification of molecular alterations characteristic of malignant thyroid nodules in the material obtained by FNA. To do that, it is necessary to know which oncogene(s) are mainly involved in thyroid cell transformation, the pathway(s) they stimulate and the mutation responsible for oncogene(s) activation. These aspects will be discussed in this chapter.

**Keywords:** BRAF, RAS oncogene, RET/PTC rearrangements, molecular diagnosis.

## INTRODUCTION

Indeterminate lesions account for nearly 20% of all FNAC, and they cannot be differentiated with respect to their benign or malignant nature, based on cytological features. In these cases, most patients undergo surgery, even though only 8-17% of them will be found to have thyroid cancer. Therefore, many patients in this category are submitted to unnecessary thyroidectomy and are exposed to the risk of surgical complications. This approach contributes to increased medical costs. The need to search for informative genetic alterations in

[*]Address correspondence to Silvia Cantara: Section of Endocrinology & Metabolism, Department of Internal Medicine, Endocrinology & Metabolism and Biochemistry, University of Siena, Siena, Italy; Email: cantara@unisi.it

this cytological category is evident, and for the first time, the revised guidelines for the management of thyroid cancer published by ATA in 2009 have provided a level C recommendation in support for molecular markers to improve the management of patients with indeterminate cytology. In this chapter, we will discuss the oncogenes that should be evaluated in fine needle aspirates, their pathogenetic mechanism and their frequency in thyroid cancer.

## RAS ONCOGENE(S)

RAS genes (H-RAS, N-RAS and K-RAS) encode four different proteins (one H-Ras, one N-Ras and two K- Ras) of approximately 21 kD, which are involved in cellular differentiation, division and cell death [1]. Each protein has a covalently attached lipid tail at the C-terminus, composed of a farnesyl, palmitol or geranylgeranyl group, which enables the Ras protein to anchor itself to cytoplasmic membrane. When Ras is inactive, it binds a GDP molecule. The Ras signaling cycle starts following an upstream stimulatory signal. Ras moves from its inactive condition to an active GTP-bound state due to guanine nucleotide exchange factor (GEF) stimulation [2]. Then, using its own intrinsic GTPase, Ras cleaves GTP, returning to its basal state. This reaction is mediated by a group of proteins called GTPase-activating proteins (GAPs) (Fig. **1**).

Ras-GAPs interaction causes an increment of approximately 1000-fold in the GTPase activity of the Ras protein, resulting in a rapid conversion from an active to an inactive form [2]. Point mutations of Ras block this cycle by inactivating the intrinsic GTPase activity (in particular by inhibiting GAP protein interaction) of Ras, maintaining the protein in its active state. Studies show that the $12^{th}$, $13^{th}$ and $61^{st}$ residues of Ras are those mainly affected by point mutations. These amino acid residues are located near the catalytic GTPase domain of Ras. Consequently, almost all substitution of these amino acids compromise GTPase function. In particular, the glycine to valine substitution at residue 12 freezes the protein in the active state, rendering the GTPase domain of Ras insensitive to inactivation by GAP.

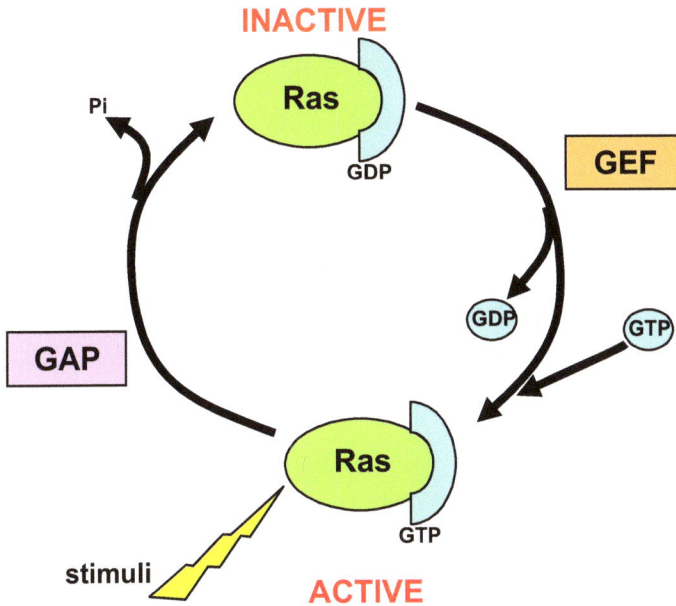

**Figure 1:** Ras activation/inactivation cycle.

Residue 61 blocks the transition state for GTP hydrolysis, reducing the rate of intrinsic Ras GTP hydrolysis to very low levels [3]. Activated Ras acts downstream through three different pathways (Fig. **2**): 1) the PI3K-Akt pathway which, inhibits Bad (implicated in apoptosis inhibition), stimulates mTOR (involved in cell growth) and inhibits GSK-3β (involved in cell proliferation) [4-6]; 2) the Raf-MEK-ERK1/2 pathway. The activation of Raf by Ras is dependent upon Raf relocalization. Once it has bound GTP, activated Ras attracts and binds Raf *via* its effector loop. Raf becomes phosphorylated and in turn it phosphorylates and activates MEK. MEK acts on another effector called ERK1/2 which proceeds to phosphorylate cytoplasmic substrates and translocates to the nucleus where it is responsible for the phosphorylation of transcription factors implicated in the immediate or delayed early gene response [7-9]; 3) Ral-GEF (Ral guanine nucleotide exchange factor) pathway. Ral A and Ral B are Ras-like proteins and share 58% sequence identity with Ras. Ral-GEF stimulates a Ral protein to move from a GDP- to a GTP-binding state. Activated Ral proteins inhibit Rho proteins such as Rac and Cdc42 involved in lamellipodia formation and cytoskeleton reorganization, respectively [10-12]. In conclusion, Ras proteins (N-, H-, or K-Ras), activating multiple control pathways at the same time, induces many of the phenotypic changes involved in neoplastic transformation. Ras mutations are found in approximately 20-50% of follicular thyroid carcinoma [13, 14], in 10% of papillary thyroid cancer (mainly the follicular variant), in poorly differentiated thyroid cancer [15-17] and in macro- and micro-follicular adenomas [18-20]. The presence of Ras mutations in malignant as well as benign lesions has led some to suggest that Ras activation may be an early event in thyroid carcinogenesis, but this hypothesis is still under debate [20, 21].

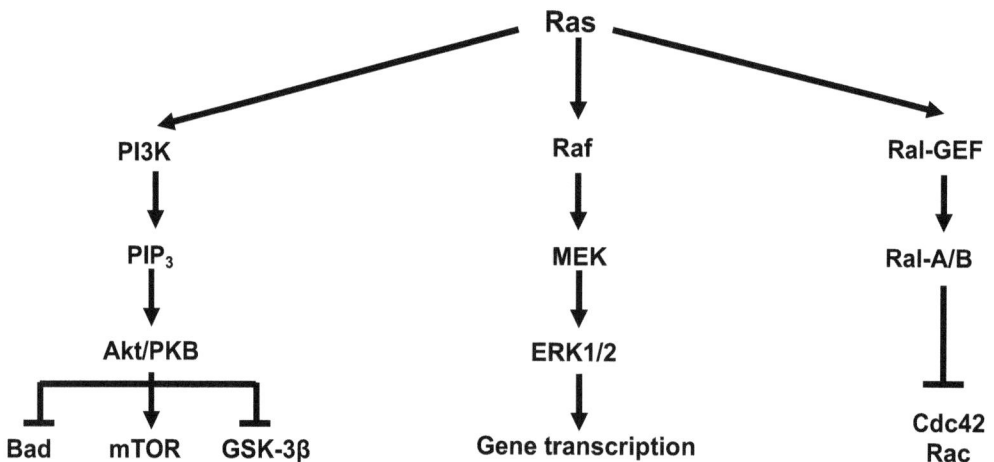

**Figure 2:** Ras signaling pathways.

## RET ONCOGENE

The Ret proto-oncogene is located at chromosome 10 (10q11.2) and encodes a tyrosine kinase cell surface receptor for members of the glial cell line-derived neurotrophic factor family such as GDNF, neurturin, artemin, and persephin [22]. These molecules activate RET *via* different glycosyl phosphatidylinositol-linked

GFRα receptors [23]. Ret gene alternative splicing results in the production of 3 different isoforms named RET51, RET43 and RET9 which contain 51, 43 and 9 amino acids in their C- terminal tail, respectively [24]. The RET51 and RET9 are the most common isoforms *in vivo* [25]. Ret protein is made up of an N-terminal extracellular domain with four cadherin-like repeats, a cysteine-rich region and nine N- glycosylation sites; a hydrophobic transmembrane domain and a cytoplasmic tyrosine kinase domain which contains 16 tyrosine residues in RET9 and 18 in RET51 [26] (Fig. **3**).

Ret activates the Raf/Mek/ERK1/2 cascade, which regulates cell proliferation, and the phosphatidylinositol 3-kinase (PI3K)/Akt signal transduction pathway, which regulates cellular survival [27, 28].

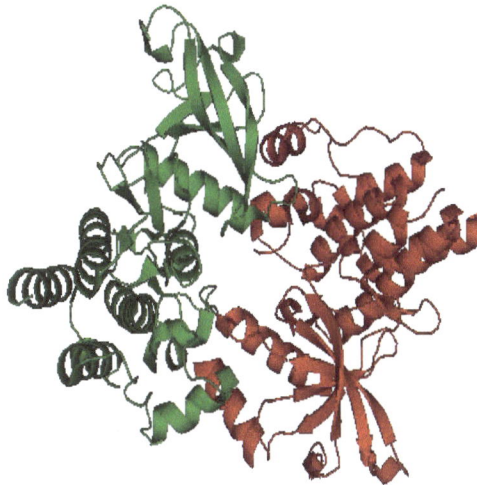

**Figure 3:** TK domain of two RET proteins (show in green and red) after receptor dimerization.

In thyroid follicular cells, Ret is normally expressed at very low levels [29]. The RET/PTC oncogenes are rearranged forms of the RET proto-oncogene found in papillary thyroid cancers (PTC) in which the Ret C-terminal domain is linked with the promoter and N-terminal domains of unrelated genes resulting in the production of constitutively active chimeric forms of Ret. Several rearrangements have been discovered between Ret and different genes: Inversion inv(10)(q11.2;q21) with H4 gene (D10S170 locus) generates the RET/CCDC6 (PTC1) oncogene; inversion inv(10)(q11.2;q11.2) with ELE1 gene generates the RET/NCOA4 (PTC3) oncogene; translocation t(10;14)(q11;q32) with GOLGA5 generates the RET/GOLGA5 (PTC5) oncogene; translocation t(8;10)(p21.3;q11.2) with PCM1 generates the PCM1/RET fusion; translocation t(6;10)(p21.3;q11.2) with RFP generates the Delta RFP/RET oncogene; translocation t(1;10)(p13;q11) with TRIM33 generates the TRIM33/RET (PTC7) oncogene; translocation t(7;10)(q32;q11) with TRIM24/TIF1 generates the TRIM24/RET (PTC6) oncogene [30]. RET/PTC rearrangements are found in approximately 20% of PTC, especially in cancer from patients exposed to ionizing radiation and in Post-Chernobyl pediatric tumors [31-35]. The most common rearrangements found in papillary thyroid cancer are RET/PTC1 and RET/PTC3.

## BRAF ONCOGENE

BRAF (v-raf murine sarcoma viral oncogene homolog B1) gene is located on chromosome 7 and encodes for an 18 exon cytoplasmic protein which is translocated to the membrane after growth factor stimulation. It is a member of the Raf kinase family of serine/threonine-specific protein kinases, along with ARAF and CRAF, and shares three conserved regions (CR1, CR2 and CR3) with them [36]. CR1, composed of 131 aa, includes the cysteine-rich domain and most of the Ras binding domain that binds RAS-GTP. CR2 has 16 aa and is rich in serine and threonine residues, including S365, an inhibitory phosphorylation site. The CR3, made up of 293 aa, contains the kinase domain, the G-loop GXGXXG motif, the activation segment and the regulatory phosphorylation sites S446, S447, D448, D449, T599 and S602 (Fig. **4**) [37, 38].

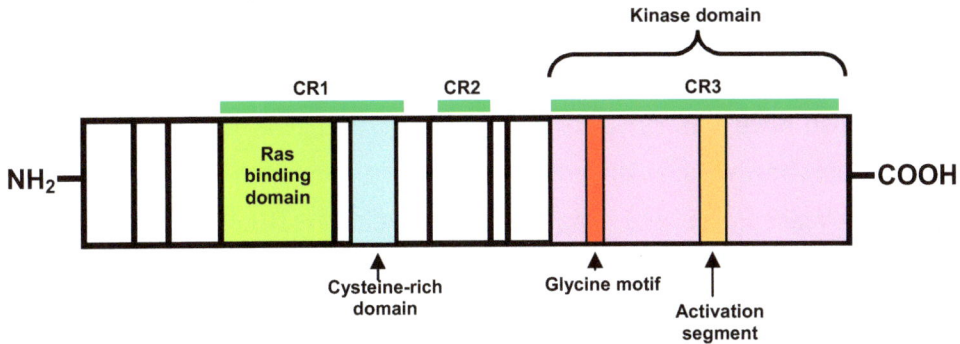

**Figure 4:** Schematic representation of the BRAF protein showing the CR1, CR2 and CR3 regions with the Ras binding domain, the cysteine rich region, the glycine motif and the activation segment.

BRAF interacts with other proteins such as HRAS, AKT, CRAF and has been demonstrated to play a role in cell growth, differentiation, and survival through ERK1/2 activation (Fig. **5**) [39, 40].

More than 30 alterations of BRAF associated with human cancers have been found, and these mutations are mostly located within the part of the gene encoding the kinase domain [41]. Among these mutations, the V600E (T1799A) resulting in a T to A transversion at position 1799 with a valine to glutamate substitution is the most common BRAF mutation, with a prevalence of approximately 45% in PTCs [18, 42-45]. The V600E mutant has a pronounced kinase activity and stimulates the MAP kinase pathway, independently from RAS protein.

X-ray crystallography [46] showed that the normal BRAF kinase domain contains the N- and C-lobes and normally adopts an inactive GDP-binding conformation. In this inactive state, the activation segment is held in an inactive conformation as a result of hydrophobic interactions with the P-loop.

Mutant BRAF (*i.e.* the V600E) changes its conformation due to the creation of favorable electrostatic interactions between the glutamate residue at position 600 and a lysine side chain of the N-lobe. As a consequence, the interaction between the P- and N-lobes is lost, allowing the protein to bind GTP. The K601E point mutation has also been described in thyroid cancer but it is less common [47]. BRAFV600E can be found in differentiated thyroid cancer as well as in poorly differentiated thyroid cancer and anaplastic thyroid cancer. BRAF protein can also be activated by a paracentric inversion of chromosome 7, resulting in the in-frame fusion between exons 1-8 of the AKAP9 gene and exons 9-18 of BRAF [48, 49]. The fused protein includes the kinase domain and lacks the auto inhibitory amino-terminal part of BRAF, resulting in an increased kinase activity. This rearrangement has been found in approximately 11% of PTC after radiation exposure and only in 1% of PTC with no history of radiation [50].

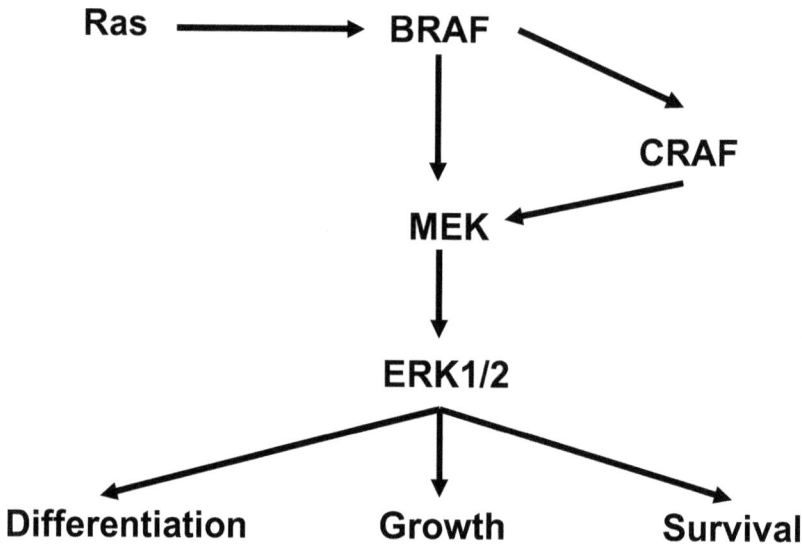

**Figure 5:** BRAF signaling pathway.

## PAX8-PPARγ REARRANGEMENTS

PAX8 (paired box 8) gene is located on chromosome 2 and is a member of the paired box (PAX) family of transcription factors [51]. The gene encodes for a nuclear protein which contains a paired box domain, an octapeptide, and a paired-type homeodomain. Five different isoforms of the protein have been described due to alternative splicing: isoform a (450 aa); isoform b (387 aa, lack exon 8); isoform c (398 aa, lack exons 7, 8); isoform d (321 aa, lack exon 8) and isoform e (287 aa, lack exons 8, 9, 10) [52].

Pax8 is found in embryonal tissues, especially in the developing thyroid gland and kidney, and it is only in these tissues that adult expression is observed [53]. The PPARγ (peroxisome proliferators-activated receptor gamma) gene is located on chromosome 3 at position p25. The encoded proteins are a group of nuclear receptor proteins that function as transcription factors regulating expression of genes involved in cellular differentiation, development, and metabolism [54]. Endogenous ligands for PPARγ are prostaglandin 2 (PGJ2). Upon activation, the receptor heterodimerizes with the retinoid X receptor (RXR) and binds to target genes in DNA consensus regions termed termed PPREs (peroxisome proliferators hormone response elements) [55]. In about 35% of follicular thyroid cancer and in a small portion of papillary thyroid cancer follicular variant, a PAX8-PPARγ rearrangement has been described [56-58]. The molecular event is represented by an interchromosomal translocation t(2;3)(q13;p25) which fuses promoter elements of PAX8 gene with most of the coding sequence of PPARγ gene.

PAX8 can break at the junction between exon 7 and exon 8, exon 8 and exon 9 or exon 7 and 9 (losing exon 8) and fuse with exon 1 of PPARγ gene (Fig. **6**) [59]. The fusion protein has also been identified in a subset of follicular adenomas (5-10%) [60].

## NTRK1 ONCOGENE

Neurotrophic tyrosine kinase, receptor, type 1 (NTRK1) gene, also named TRK, is located on the q arm of chromosome 1 (1q21-22) and encodes for a member of the neurotrophic tyrosine kinase receptor (NTKR) family [61]. This kinase is a membrane-bound receptor that, upon neurotrophin binding (*i.e.* NGF), phosphorylates itself and members of the MAPK pathway, leading to cell differentiation and allowing the formation of specific sensory neuron subtypes [62]. In papillary thyroid cancer, chimeric proteins (TRK rearrangements) have been identified, with constitutive and ectopic enzymatic activity due to somatic rearrangements juxtaposing the tyrosine kinase domain to 5 '-end sequences of unrelated loci [63, 64]. To date, there are at least three genes known to be involved in TRK rearrangements: TPM3 located at 1q22-23, TGF located at 3q11-12 and TPR located at 1q25. TRK is a rearranged protein involving NTRK1 and TPM3; TRK1 and TRK2 are chimeric proteins involving NTRK1 and TPR and TRK3 is the rearranged product of NTKR1 and TGF. The frequency of these events in papillary thyroid cancer is approximately 10% [65].

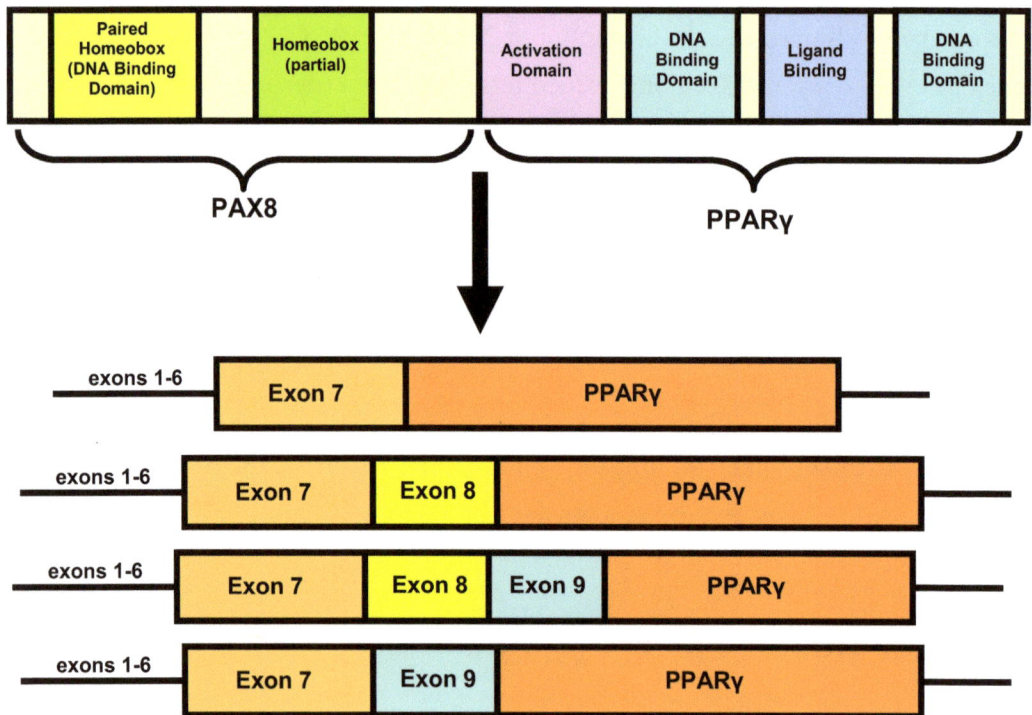

**Figure 6:** Upper part of the figure: generic rearrangement between PAX8 and PPARγ genes. Lower part of the figure: several rearrangements showing different exons of PAX8 gene that can be involved in the formation of the chimeric protein.

# P53 POINT MUTATIONS

p53 is encoded by the TP53 gene located on the short arm of chromosome 17 (17p13.1). The gene is highly conserved in vertebrates, specially with respect to five regions in the coding sequence predominantly in exons 2, 5, 6, 7 and 8. The protein is composed by 393 aminoacids divided into 7 domains: an N-terminus transcription-activation domain (TAD), which activates transcription factors; an activation domain 2 (AD2) important for apoptotic activity; a proline rich domain; a DNA-binding site; a domain involved in nuclear localization; a site responsible for p53 tetramerization and a C-terminal domain which contributes to regulate DNA binding activity of the central site. P53 induces cell growth arrest, contributes to DNA damage repair, plays a role in apoptosis, inhibits angiogenesis and contributes to genomic stability. P53 point mutations impair its transcriptional activity, and occur in 55% of ATCs [66].

# CONFLICT OF INTEREST

The author confirms that she has no conflicts of interest.

# ACKNOWLEDGEMENTS

None Declared.

# REFERENCES

[1]     Barbacid M. Ras genes. Annu Rev. Biochem. 1987, 56:779-827.
[2]     Vetter IR, Wittinghofer A. The guanine nucleotide-binding switch in three dimensions. Science 2001, 294:1299-304.
[3]     Roskoski R Jr. RAF protein-serine/threonine kinases: structure and regulation. Biochem Biophys Res Commun. 2010, 399:313-7.
[4]     Viglietto G, Amodio N, Malanga D, Scrima M, De Marco C. Contribution of PKB/AKT signaling to thyroid cancer. Front Biosci. 2011, 16:1461-87.
[5]     Franke TF, Yang SI, Chan TO, Datta K, Kazlauskas A, Morrison DK, Kaplan DR, Tsichlis PN. The protein kinase encoded by the Akt proto-oncogene is a target of the PDGF-activated phosphatidylinositol 3-kinase. Cell 1995, 81:727-36.

[6]     Mendoza MC, Er EE, Blenis J. The Ras-ERK and PI3K-mTOR pathways: cross-talk and compensation. Trends Biochem Sci. 2011, 36:320-8.

[7]     Kolch W, Kotwaliwale A, Vass K, Janosch P. The role of Raf kinases in malignant transformation. Expert Rev Mol Med. 2002, 4:1-18.

[8]     Williams NG, Paradis H, Agarwal S, Charest DL, Pelech SL, Roberts TM. Raf-1 and p21v-ras cooperate in the activation of mitogen-activated protein kinase. PNAS 1993, 90:5772-6.

[9]     Dent P, Wu J, Romero G, Vincent LA, Castle D, Sturgill TW. Activation of the mitogen-activated protein kinase pathway in Triton X-100 disrupted NIH-3T3 cells by p21 ras and *in vitro* by plasma membranes from NIH 3T3 cells. Mol Biol Cell. 1993, 4:483-93. Erratum in: Mol Biol Cell 6:1261.

[10]    Martin TD, Samuel JC, Routh ED, Der CJ, Yeh JJ. Activation and involvement of Ral GTPases in colorectal cancer. Cancer Res. 2011, 71:206-15.

[11]    Kidd AR 3rd, Snider JL, Martin TD, Graboski SF, Der CJ, Cox AD. Ras-related small GTPases RalA and RalB regulate cellular survival after ionizing radiation. Int J Radiat Oncol Biol Phys. 2010, 78:205-12.

[12]    Poghosyan Z, Wynford-Thomas D. Analysis of Ras transformation of human thyroid epithelial cells. Methods Enzymol. 2006, 407:648-60.

[13]    Esapa CT, Johnson SJ, Kendall-Taylor P. Prevalence of Ras mutations in thyroid neoplasia. Clinical Endocrinoly 1999, 50:529-535.

[14]    Vasko V, Ferrand M, Di Cristofaro J, Carayon P, Henry JF, de Micco C. Specific pattern of RAS oncogene mutations in follicular thyroid tumors. JCEM. 2003, 88:2745-52.

[15]    Suárez HG, Du Villard JA, Caillou B, Schlumberger M, Tubiana M, Parmentier C, Monier R. Detection of activated ras oncogenes in human thyroid carcinomas. Oncogene 1988, 2:403-6.

[16]    Namba H, Rubin SA, Fagin JA. Point mutations of ras oncogenes are an early event in thyroid tumorigenesis. Mol Endocrinol. 1990, 4:1474-9.

[17]    Zhu Z, Gandhi M, Nikiforova MN, Fischer AH, Nikiforov YE. Molecular profile and clinical-pathologic features of the follicular variant of papillary thyroid carcinoma. An unusually high prevalence of ras mutations. Am J Clin Pathol. 2003, 120:71-7.

[18]    Cantara S, Capezzone M, Marchisotta S, Capuano S, Busonero G, Toti P, Di Santo A, Caruso G, Carli AF, Brilli L, Montanaro A, Pacini F. Impact of proto-oncogene mutation detection in cytological specimens from thyroid nodules improves the diagnostic accuracy of cytology. JCEM 2010, 95:1365-9.

[19]    Palos-Paz F, Perez-Guerra O, Cameselle-Teijeiro J, Rueda-Chimeno C, Barreiro-Morandeira F, Lado-Abeal J; Galician Group for the Study of Toxic Multinodular Goitre, Araujo Vilar D, Argueso R, Barca O, Botana M, Cabezas-Agrícola JM, Catalina P, Dominguez Gerpe L, Fernandez T, Mato A, Nuño A, Penin M, Victoria B. Prevalence of mutations in TSHR, GNAS, PRKAR1A and RAS genes in a large series of toxic thyroid

adenomas from Galicia, an iodine-deficient area in NW Spain. Eur J Endocrinol. 2008, 159:623-31.

[20]  Vasko VV, Gaudart J, Allasia C, Savchenko V, Di Cristofaro J, Saji M, Ringel MD, De Micco C. Thyroid follicular adenomas may display features of follicular carcinoma and follicular variant of papillary carcinoma. Eur J Endocrinol. 2004, 151:779-86.

[21]  Wynford-Thomas D. Origin and progression of thyroid epithelial tumours: cellular and molecular mechanisms. Horm Res. 1997, 47:145-57.

[22]  Ceccherini I, Bocciardi R, Luo Y, Pasini B, Hofstra R, Takahashi M, Romeo G. Exon structure and flanking intronic sequences of the human RET proto-oncogene. Biochem Biophys Res Commun. 1993, 96:1288-95.

[23]  Airaksinen MS, Titievsky A, Saarma M. GDNF family neurotrophic factor signaling: four masters, one servant?. Mol. Cell Neurosci. 1999, 13:313–25.

[24]  Myers SM, Eng C, Ponder BA, Mulligan LM. Characterization of RET proto-oncogene 3' splicing variants and polyadenylation sites: a novel C-terminus for RET. Oncogene 1995, 11:2039-45.

[25]  Hickey JG, Myers SM, Tian X, Zhu SJ, V Shaw JL, Andrew SD, Richardson DS, Brettschneider J, Mulligan LM. RET-mediated gene expression pattern is affected by isoform but not oncogenic mutation. Genes Chromosomes Cancer. 2009, 48:429-40.

[26]  Knowles PP, Murray-Rust J, Kjaer S, Scott RP, Hanrahan S, Santoro M, Ibáñez CF, McDonald NQ. Structure and chemical inhibition of the RET tyrosine kinase domain. J Biol Chem. 2006, 281:33577-87.

[27]  Zbuk KM and Eng C. Cancer phenomics: RET and PTEN as illustrative models. Nat Rev Cancer. 2007, 7:35-45.

[28]  Liu R, Liu D, Trink E, Bojdani E, Ning G, Xing M. The Akt-specific inhibitor MK2206 selectively inhibits thyroid cancer cells harboring mutations that can activate the PI3K/Akt pathway. J Clin Endocrinol Metab. 2011, 96:E577-85.

[29]  Powers JF, Brachold JM, Tischler AS. Ret protein expression in adrenal medullary hyperplasia and pheochromocytoma. Endocr. Pathol. 2003, 14:351-61.

[30]  Zitzelsberger H, Bauer V, Thomas G and Unger K. Molecular rearrangements in papillary thyroid carcinomas. Clinica Chimica Acta 2010, 411:301-8.

[31]  Bongarzone I, Monzini N, Borrello MG, Carcano C, Ferraresi G, Arighi E, Mondellini P, Della Porta G, Pierotti MA Molecular characterization of a thyroid tumor-specific transforming sequence formed by the fusion of ret tyrosine kinase and the regulatory subunit RI alpha of cyclic AMP-dependent protein kinase A. Molecular and Cellular Biology 1993, 13:358–366.

[32]  Santoro M, Dathan NA, Berlingieri MT, Bongarzone I, Paulin C, Grieco M, Pierotti MA, Vecchio G, Fusco A. Molecular characterization of RET/PTC3; a novel rearranged version of the RET proto-oncogene in a human thyroid papillary carcinoma. Oncogene 1994, 9:509–516.

[33] Elisei R, Romei C, Vorontsova T, Cosci B, Veremeychik V, Kuchinskaya E, Basolo F, Demidchik EP, Miccoli P, Pinchera A, Pacini F. RET/PTC rearrangements in thyroid nodules: studies in irradiated and not irradiated, malignant and benign thyroid lesions in children and adults. Journal of Clinical Endocrinology and Metabolism 2001, 86:3211–3216.

[34] Tuttle RM, Lukes Y, Onstad L, Lushnikov E, Abrosimov A, Troshin V, Tsyb A, Davis S, Kopecky KJ, Francis G. ret/PTC activation is not associated with individual radiation dose estimates in a pilot study of neoplastic thyroid nodules arising in Russian children and adults exposed to Chernobyl fallout. Thyroid 2008, 18:839-46.

[35] Nikiforov YE. Radiation-induced thyroid cancer: what we have learned from chernobyl. Endocr Pathol. 2006, 17:307-17.

[36] Sithanandam G, Druck T, Cannizzaro LA, Leuzzi G, Huebner K, Rapp UR. B-raf and a B-raf pseudogene are located on 7q in man. Oncogene 1992, 7:795–9.

[37] see: http://atlasgeneticsoncology.org

[38] Kumagai A, Namba H, Takakura S, Inamasu E, Saenko VA, Ohtsuru A, Yamashita S. No evidence of ARAF, CRAF and MET mutations in BRAFT1799A negative human papillary thyroid carcinoma. Endocr J. 2006, 53:615-20.

[39] Mitsutake N, Miyagishi M, Mitsutake S, Akeno N, Mesa C Jr, Knauf JA, Zhang L, Taira K, Fagin JA. BRAF mediates RET/PTC-induced mitogen-activated protein kinase activation in thyroid cells: functional support for requirement of the RET/PTC-RAS-BRAF pathway in papillary thyroid carcinogenesis. Endocrinology. 2006, 147:1014-9.

[40] Brummer, T. B-Raf signaling. Essay for the second edition of the Encyclopedia of Cancer (Springer). Edited by Manfred Schwab, 2008.

[41] Davies H, Bignell GR, Cox C, Stephens P, Edkins S, Clegg S, Teague J, Woffendin H, Garnett MJ, Bottomley W, Davis N, Dicks E, Ewing R, Floyd Y, Gray K, Hall S, Hawes R, Hughes J, Kosmidou V, Menzies A, Mould C, Parker A, Stevens C, Watt S, Hooper S, Wilson R, Jayatilake H, Gusterson BA, Cooper C, Shipley J, Hargrave D, Pritchard-Jones K, Maitland N, Chenevix-Trench G, Riggins GJ, Bigner DD, Palmieri G, Cossu A, Flanagan A, Nicholson A, Ho JW, Leung SY, Yuen ST, Weber BL, Seigler HF, Darrow TL, Paterson H, Marais R, Marshall CJ, Wooster R, Stratton MR, Futreal PA. Mutation of the BRAF gene in human cancer. Nature 2002, 417:949-54.

[42] Xing M. BRAF mutation in thyroid cancer. Endocrine-related Cancer. 2005, 12:245-262.

[43] Durante C, Tallini G, Puxeddu E, Sponziello M, Moretti S, Ligorio C, Cavaliere A, Rhoden KJ, Verrienti A, Maranghi M, Giacomelli L, Russo D, Filetti S. BRAF V600E mutation and expression of proangiogenic molecular markers in papillary thyroid carcinomas. Eur J Endocrinol. 2011, 165:455-463.

[44] Proietti A, Giannini R, Ugolini C, Miccoli M, Fontanini G, Di Coscio G, Romani R, Berti P, Miccoli P, Basolo F. BRAF status of follicular variant of papillary thyroid carcinoma and its relationship to its clinical and cytological features. Thyroid. 2010, 20:1263-70.

[45]   Elisei R, Ugolini C, Viola D, Lupi C, Biagini A, Giannini R, Romei C, Miccoli P, Pinchera A, Basolo F. BRAF(V600E) mutation and outcome of patients with papillary thyroid carcinoma: a 15-year median follow-up study. J. Clin. Endocrinol. Metab. 2008, 93:3943–9.

[46]   see: http://hdl.handle.net/2381/7858

[47]   Xing M. BRAF mutation in papillary thyroid cancer: pathogenic role, molecular bases, and clinical implications. Endocr Rev. 2007, 28:742-62.

[48]   Ciampi R, Knauf JA, Kerler R, Gandhi M, Zhu Z, Nikiforova MN, Rabes HM, Fagin JA, Nikiforov YE. J Clin Invest. 2005, 115:94-101.

[49]   Gandhi M, Evdokimova V, Nikiforov YE. Mechanisms of chromosomal rearrangements in solid tumors: the model of papillary thyroid carcinoma. Mol Cell Endocrinol. 2010, 321:36-43.

[50]   Lee JH, Lee ES, Kim YS, Won NH, Chae YS. BRAF mutation and AKAP9 expression in sporadic papillary thyroid carcinomas. Pathology. 2006, 38:201-4.

[51]   Stapleton P, Weith A, Urbánek P, Kozmik Z, Busslinger M. Chromosomal localization of seven PAX genes and cloning of a novel family member, PAX-9. Nat Genet. 1993, 3:292-8.

[52]   Kozmik Z, Kurzbauer R, Dorfler P, Busslinger M. Alternative splicing of Pax-8 gene transcripts is developmentally regulated and generates isoforms with different transactivation properties. Mol Cell Biol. 1993, 13:6024-35.

[53]   Mansouri A, Hallonet M, Gruss P. Pax genes and their roles in cell differentiation and development. Curr Opin Cell Biol. 1996, 8:851-7.

[54]   Michalik L, Auwerx J, Berger JP, Chatterjee VK, Glass CK, Gonzalez FJ, Grimaldi PA, Kadowaki T, Lazar MA, O'Rahilly S, Palmer CN, Plutzky J, Reddy JK, Spiegelman BM, Staels B, Wahli W. International Union of Pharmacology. LXI. Peroxisome proliferator-activated receptors. Pharmacol. Rev. 2006, 58:726-41.

[55]   Marlow LA, Reynolds LA, Cleland AS, Cooper SJ, Gumz ML, Kurakata S, Fujiwara K, Zhang Y, Sebo T, Grant C, McIver B, Wadsworth JT, Radisky DC, Smallridge RC, Copland JA. Reactivation of suppressed RhoB is a critical step for the inhibition of anaplastic thyroid cancer growth. Cancer Res. 2009, 69:1536–44.

[56]   Kroll TG, Sarraf P, Pecciarini L, Chen CJ, Mueller E, Spiegelman BM and Fletcher JA. PAX8-PPARgamma1 fusion oncogene in human thyroid carcinoma. Science 2000, 289:1357–1360

[57]   Nikiforova MN, Biddinger PW, Caudill CM, Kroll TG, Nikiforov YE. PAX8-PPARgamma rearrangement in thyroid tumors: RT-PCR and immunohistochemical analyses. American Journal of Surgical Pathology 2002, 26:1016–1023.

[58]   Castro P, Rebocho AP, Soares RJ, Magalhaes J, Roque L, Trovisco V, Vieira de Castro I, Cardoso-de-Oliveira M, Fonseca E, Soares P and Sobrinho-Simões M. PAX8-PPARgamma

rearrangement is frequently detected in the follicular variant of papillary thyroid carcinoma. Journal of Clinical Endocrinology and Metabolism 2006, 91:213–220

[59]  Hibi Y, Nagaya T, Kambe F, Imai T, Funahashi H, Nakao A, Seo H. Is thyroid follicular cancer in Japanese caused by a specific t(2; 3)(q13; p25) translocation generating Pax8-PPAR gamma fusion mRNA? Endocr J. 2004, 51:361-6.

[60]  Marques AR, Espadinha C, Catarino AL, Moniz S, Pereira T, Sobrinho LG and Leite V Expression of PAX8-PPAR gamma 1 rearrangements in both follicular thyroid carcinomas and adenomas. Journal of Clinical Endocrinology and Metabolism 2002, 87:3947–3952.

[61]  see: http://www.genecards.org/cgi-bin/carddisp.pl?gene=NTRK1

[62]  Huang EJ, Reichardt LF. Trk receptors: roles in neuronal signal transduction. Annu. Rev. Biochem. 2003, 72:609–642.

[63]  Pierotti MA, Greco A. Oncogenic rearrangements of the NTRK1/NGF receptor. Cancer Lett. 2006, 232:90-8.

[64]  Greco A, Miranda C, Pierotti MA. Rearrangements of NTRK1 gene in papillary thyroid carcinoma. Mol Cell Endocrinol. 2010, 321:44-9.

[65]  Greco A, Miranda C, Pagliardini S, Fusetti L, Bongarzone I, Pierotti MA. Chromosome 1 rearrangements involving the genes TPR and NTRK1 produce structurally different thyroid-specific TRK oncogenes. Genes Chromosomes Cancer. 1997, 19:112-23.

[66]  Smallridge RC, Marlow LA, Copland JA. Anaplastic thyroid cancer: molecular pathogenesis and emerging therapies. Endocr Relat Cancer. 2009, 16:17–44.

# CHAPTER 4

## Methods for Oncogene Analysis in Thyroid FNAC

**Silvia Cantara***

*Section of Endocrinology & Metabolism, Department of Internal Medicine, Endocrinology & Metabolism and Biochemistry, University of Siena, Siena, Italy*

**Abstract:** Several oncogenes are involved in the development of thyroid cancer. In the last 10 years, different techniques have been applied to study point mutations and genetic rearrangements. Some of them have been used only on thyroid specimens and need to be tested on FNAC material. Generally, these modifications can be studied by various PCR-based techniques, and results depend on the quality and quantity of the starting material. By carefully selecting the appropriate methods, researchers have demonstrated that the detection of genetic alterations is feasible in a FNAC samples. This may refine the diagnosis of thyroid cancer, especially for those samples which are deemed cytologically inadequate.

**Keywords:** Mutation detection, PCR, nested PCR, real time PCR, Southern blot, molecular techniques.

## INTRODUCTION

Genetic modifications, such as point mutations and rearrangements, can be evaluated in a tissue sample applying molecular techniques. The use of a FNAC sample is not simple, because the starting material may be inadequate in terms of quantity and quality. Despite the low amounts of RNA obtained, useful information can be generated by applying highly specific and sensible techniques. Several diagnostic methods using real time PCR technology or allele-specific

---

*****Address correspondence to Silvia Cantara:** Section of Endocrinology & Metabolism, Department of Internal Medicine, Endocrinology & Metabolism and Biochemistry, University of Siena, Siena, Italy; Email: cantara@unisi.it

oligonucelotides PCR have been developed, with encouraging results. In this chapter, methods to study genetic alterations responsible for the development of thyroid cancer are proposed.

## RNA EXTRACTION AND QUALITY ASSESSMENT

RNA is a nucleic acid, but differs from DNA in three ways. First, RNA is, generally, a single-stranded molecule and has shorter chains of nucleotides. Second, the complementary base to adenine is not thymine but uracil. Third, while DNA contains deoxyribose, RNA contains ribose with a hydroxyl group attached to the pentose ring. These hydroxyl groups render RNA more susceptible to hydrolysis and, as a result, RNA is less stable than DNA. This notion needs to be taken into consideration when the FNAC sampe is processed for RNA extraction. The FNAC sample should be collected in a microcentrifuge tube (1.5 ml) containing a RNA stabilizer and eventually stored until use at -20°C or -80°C. At the moment of the extraction, the reagent should be removed by centrifugation, the FNAC material recovered and the RNA extracted using commercial kits. It is optimal to use kits for total RNA extraction. RNA concentration and purification yield can be assessed spectrophotometrically [1] calculating the ratio of absorbance values at 260nm *vs.* 280nm. This value is commonly used to assess protein contamination of nucleic acid solutions, since proteins (in particular, the aromatic amino acids) absorb light at 280nm [2]. For pure RNA, $A_{260/280}$ is approximately 2. Another method to verify the quantity and quality of isolated RNA is to amplify genes such as BRAF, RAS or GAPDH by real time PCR, and to consider the sample satisfactory when the amplification cycle threshold (Ct) is less than 35 cycles [3]. To perform this type of analysis, RNA needs to be retro-transcribed into complementary DNA (cDNA). Once the quality and quantity of the material is verified, the presence of thyroid cells in the sample should be confirmed. This can be done by amplifying a marker of thyroidal cells (*i.e.* thyroperoxidase, TSH receptor) [1] by PCR, or by real time PCR quantification of a marker of epithelial cells (*i.e.* KRT7) *vs.* GAPDH [3]. The difference in amplification of more than 3.5 cycles corresponds to approximately 10% of thyroid epithelial cells within the sample [3].

## METHODS BASED ON DNA

Another possibility is to isolate DNA from a FNAC sample. In this case, the extraction yields more nucleic acid and of better quality. The presence of thyroidal cells and the A260/280 ratio still needs to be verified. The target ratio is approximately 1.8. When the quantity of DNA is low, DNA can be amplified using specific kits for whole genome amplification, rendering the sample adequate for the analysis. DNA can be used for evaluation of rearrangement when the recombining intron size is adequate for PCR amplification. In other cases, the use of RNA is recommended.

## METHODS FOR THE ANALYSIS OF RAS POINT MUTATIONS

1) <u>PCR:</u> To identify RAS mutations (H-, K-, and NRAS) codons 12, 13 and 61 should be amplified by PCR, either from DNA or cDNA [1, 4, 5]. Generally, 200 ng of template are added to a mix containing 200 nM of each primer, 200 μM of dNTPs, 1.5-2.5 mM $MgCl_2$ and 0.25-1.25 U Taq Polymerase. According to primer characteristics (*i.e.* content of GC, length, melting temperature) annealing temperature can vary from 50°C to 65°C for 35-40 cycles. Examples of primers are listed in Table **1**. Next, the PCR products are submitted to electrophoresis on a 2-3% agarose gel, and resolved according to product length. The presence of point mutations is then verified with direct sequencing directly, or after a previous step with Denaturing High Performance Liquid Chromatography (DHPLC) which allows detection of unknown genetic mutations and single nucleotide polymorphisms (SNPs) based on DNA heteroduplex formation and separation of heteroduplex from homoduplex molecular species [6].

**Table 1:** Primers for RAS point mutation identification by PCR [1, 4, 5]

| Gene | Primers | Template |
|------|---------|----------|
| HRAS | F:5'CCTGAGGAGCGATGACGGAATA3' <br> R:5'TCCGAGTCCTTCACCCGTTTGA3' | cDNA |
| NRAS | F: 5'CCCGGTCTGTGGTCCTAAATC3' <br> R: 'CGCCTGTCCTCATGTATTGGTCT3' | cDNA |
| KRAS | F:5'GCCATTTCGGACTGGGAGCGAG3' <br> R: 'GCCCTCCCCAGTCCTCATGTACT3' | cDNA |
| HRAS 12/13 | F: 5'ATGACGGAATATAAGCTGGT3' <br> R: 5'CTCTATAGTGGGGTCGTATT3' | DNA |
| HRAS 61 | F: 5'AGGTGGTCATTGATGGGGAG3' <br> R: 5'AGGAAGCCCTCCCCGGTGCG3' | DNA |
| NRAS 12/13 | F: 5'ATGACTGAGTACAAACTGGT3' <br> R: 5'CTCTATGGTGGGATCATATT3' | DNA |
| NRAS 61 | F: 5'TCTTACAGAAAACAAGTGGT3' <br> R: 5'GTAGAGGTTAATATCCGCAA3' | DNA |
| KRAS 12/13 | F: 5'GGCCTGCTGAAAATGACTGAA3' <br> R: 5'GGTCCTGCACCAGTAATATGC3' | DNA |
| KRAS 61 | F:5'CAGGATTCCTACAGGAAGCAAGTAG3' <br> R: 5'CACAAAGAAAGCCCTCCCCA3' | DNA |

2) <u>Real time PCR:</u> RAS mutations can also be analyzed with real-time PCR and fluorescence curve analysis [3, 5, 7, 8]. This method is based on rapid-cycle PCR amplification of the locus containing the mutated hot spot using a pair of primers and two fluorescently labelled oligonucleotide probes that hybridize adjacent to one another, so that one fluorophore functions as the donor and another as the acceptor which emits at a specific wavelength [9]. Examples of primers are reported in Table **2**.

**Table 2:** Primers for RAs point mutation identification by real time PCR [6]

| Gene | Primers and probes |
|------|--------------------|
| NRAS 12/13 | 5'-GCT GGT GTG AAA TGA CTG AG-3'<br>5'-GAT GAT CCG ACA AGT GAG AG-3'<br>5'-TTG GAG CAG GTG GTG TTG-fluorescein-3'<br>5'-LC-Red 640-GAA AAG CGC ACT GAC AAT CCA GCT AAT CCA GAA CCA-phosphate-3' |
| NRAS 61 | 5'-CCT GTT TGT TGG ACA TAC TG-3'<br>5'-CCT GTA GAG GTT AAT ATC CG-3'<br>5'-CCT GTC CTC ATG TAT TGG TCT CTC ATG GCA CT-fluorescein-3'<br>LC-Red 705-TAC TCT TCT TGT CCA GCT GT-phosphate-3' |
| HRAS 12/13 | 5'-TGA GGA GCG ATG ACG GAA-3'<br>5'-GCG CTA GGC TCA CCT CTA T-3'<br>5'-AGC TGG ATG GTC AGC GCA CTC TTG CCC-fluorescein-3'<br>5'-LC Red640-CAC CGC CGG CGC CCA C-phosphate-3' |
| HRAS 61 | 5'-GTC CTC CTG CAG GAT TCC TA-3'<br>5'-ATG GCA AAC ACA CAC AGG AA-3'<br>5'-GAT ACC GCC GGC CAG GAG GA-fluorescein-3'<br>5'-LC Red640-TAC AGC GCCATG CGG GAC CAG T-phosphate-3' |
| KRAS 12/13 | 5'-AAG GCC TGC TGA AAA TGA CTG-3'<br>5'-GGT CCT GCA CCA GTA ATA TGC A-3'<br>5'-CGT CCA CAA AAT GAT TCT GAA TTA GCT GTA TCG TCA AGG CAC T-fluorescein-3'<br>5'-LC Red640-TGC CTA CGC CAC CAG CTC CAA-phosphate-3' |
| KRAS 61 | 5'-AGG ATT CCT ACA GGA AGC AAG TAG-3'<br>5'-CCC TCC CCA GTC CTC ATG-3'<br>5'-TGC ACT GTA CTC CTC TTG ACC TGC T-fluorescein-3'<br>5'-LC Red705-TCG AGA ATA TCC AAG AGA CAG GTT TCT CCA-phosphate-3' |

3)  <u>High Resolution Melt (HRM) analysis:</u> This is a powerful technique for the detection of point mutations in double-stranded DNA samples. The technique is based on the use of fluorescent dyes that release high fluorescence intensity when they are bound to double-stranded DNA. The melting temperature of the amplicon at which the two DNA strands come apart is entirely predictable and depends on the sequence of the DNA bases. A homozygous wild type sample always has the

same melting profile. In the presence of point mutations, the melt curve differs. The power of HRM is the ability to monitor this process in "high resolution" and, thus, it is possible to accurately identify the presence of a point mutation even in case of a small amount of starting material or a small percentage of mutated cells in the sample [10, 11].

## Final Suggestions

To study RAS point mutations, classical PCR can be really effective especially when followed by DHPLC and/or sequencing. Nevertheless, it is worth noting that the new HRM technique should be considered by every genetic analysis laboratory, especially those routinely performing these diagnostic tests. HRM is 10 times more sensitive compared to direct sequencing, allowing a correct interpretation from samples in which there are very few mutated cells. In these samples, the heterozygous mutation is often confused with signal noise when analyzed by electropherogram. Moreover, HRM is highly reproducible.

## METHODS FOR THE STUDY OF RET REARRANGEMENTS

1) <u>Nested PCR</u>: This method increases the specificity of DNA amplification, by reducing background due to non-specific amplification. Two sets of primers are used in two successive PCRs. In the first reaction, one pair of primers is used to generate DNA products, which, in addition to the intended target, may still consist of non-specifically amplified DNA fragments. The product(s) are then used in a second PCR with a set of primers whose binding sites are completely or partially different from and located 3' of each of the primers used in the first reaction. For RET/PTC1 and RET/PTC3 rearrangements, nested PCR can be applied [12] with forward primers designed in the 5' regions of H4 and Ele1 for RET/PTC1 and RET/PTC3, respectively, and reverse primers in the TK domain of RET for both rearrangements. In this case, at least 500 ng of cDNA

have to be amplified in a mixture containing 2.5 mM MgCl2 and 0.5 mM each primers (Table **3**) for 35 cycles with annealing temperatures of 68° C for RET/PTC1 and 60° C for RET/PTC3. After this first step, 1:10 PCR products need to be nested amplified with the same cycling conditions using primers reported in Table **3**.

**Table 3:** Primers for RET/PTC rearrangements [1, 12]

| RET/PTC1 F | 5'-AGCGCCAGCGAGAGCGACACG-3' |
|---|---|
| RET/PTC3 F | 5'-AGACCTTGGAGAACAGTCAG-3' |
| RET/PRC R | 5'-TACCCTGCTCTGCCTTTCAGATGG-3' |
| RET/PTC1 nested F | 5'-GTCGGGGGGCATTGTCATCT-3' |
| RET/PTC1 nested R | 5'-AGTTCTTCCGAGGGAATTCC-3' |
| RET/PTC3 nested F | 5'-AGACCTTGGAGAACAGTCAG-3' |
| RET/PTC3 nested R | 5'-AGTTCTTCCAGAGGAATTCC-3' |

2)  <u>PCR and Southern blot</u>: PCR products obtained by first PCR (for primers see Table **3**) can be verified by southern blot using specific probes such as: RET/PTC1 5'-GGCACTGCAGGAGGAGAACCGC-GA-3'; RET/PTC3 5'-GTCGGTGCTGGGTATGTAAGGA-3'. Briefly, gels should be washed three times with water to remove ethidium bromide and then rinsed for 45 min (room temperature) with a solution containing 0.5 M NaOH and 1.5 M NaCl. After, gels should be washed twice with water and then with a solution containing 0.5 M Tris-HCl and 1.5 M NaCl (45 min, room temperature). Then, DNA needs to be transferred onto a nylon membrane with 10X SSC. To block DNA, membranes must be twice exposed to an UV source at 1200 mJ and then washed in 2X SSC. Each filter have to be then hybridized with a probe and signals detected [1, 13, 14]. Other authors [15, 16] use classical PCR as the only detection method for the

analysis of RET rearrangements in FNAC samples with excellent results.

3) <u>RET/PTCX</u>: A generic rearrangement for RET is called RET/PTCX. To perform a screening for RET/PTCX samples should be analyzed for the expression of tyrosine kinase (TK) and extracellular (EC) domains using, for examples, the following primers: EC F 5'-GGCGGCCCAAGTGTGCCGAACTT-3'; EC R 5'-CCCAGGCCG-CCACACTCCTCACA-3', TK F 5'-TGGTTCTTGGAAAAACTCT-AG-3'; TK R 5'-CTGCAGGCCCCATACAATTT-3'. Only samples showing TK expression not associated with EC are considered positive for rearrangement. Thermal cycling conditions include an initial step (94° C for 10 min) followed by 35 cycles at 60° C and a final extension (72° C for 10 min). Southern blot can be used also in this case with specific probes (*i.e.* TK 5'-ACGCAAAGTGATG-TATGGTCT-3'; EC 5'-GTAACAGTGGAGGGGTCATATG-3') (1, 13, 15). Also for EC and TK amplification, not all authors perform a post PCR analysis [16].

4) <u>Real time PCR</u>: RET/PTC1 and RET/PTC3 rearrangements can be also verified by Q-RT-PCR. In a final volume of 20 µl we amplify 1 µg of cDNA in a mix containing 200 nM final concentration of specific primers and 100 nM of probes. Primers forward and probes are as follows: RET/PTC1 F 5'-CGCGACCTGCGCAAA-3', RET/PTC3 F 5'-CCCCAGGACTGGCTTACCC-3', PTC1 probe 5'-CAAGCGTAACCATCGAGGATCCAAA-3', PTC3 probe 5'-AAAGCAGACCTTGGAGAACAGTCAG-3'. For both fragments, primer reverse is: RET/PTC R 5'-CAAGTTCTTCCGAGGGAAT-TCC-3'. To verify the presence of non-rearranged RET can be used the following primers and probe: RET F 5'-TGCTTCTGCGAGCCC-

3', RET R 5'-ATCACCGTGCGGCACAG-3', RET probe 5'-CATCCAGGATCCACTGTGCA-3'. Thermal cycling profile is 3 min at 95° C followed by 15 sec at 95° C and 1 min at 60° C for 45 cycles [8].

## Final Suggestions

In 2006, Zhu *et al.* published a paper in which they compared different methodologies to study RET/PTC rearrangements [17]. They found that PCR was able to correctly identify RET/PTC rearrangements in 14/65 tumors and that, if PCR was followed by Southern blot, the number of positive cases was raised to 26/65. Real time PCR diagnosed 12/65 cancers and Southern blot alone diagnosed 11/65 cases. The results were greatly influenced by the content of positive-cells in the starting material. For the detection of RET/PTC rearrangements, the authors recommend not using highly sensitive nonquantitative methods, in order to avoid the detection of carcinomas with low RET/PTC rearrangements, which seem to have doubtful biological significance [18, 19].

Whatever method applied, it is recommended to use positive controls in each experiment such as transfected cells (*i.e.* TPC1 cell carried the RET/PTC1 rearrangement) or cloned vectors [16].

## METHODS FOR THE ANALYSIS OF BRAF POINT MUTATION

1) <u>PCR</u>: To identify BRAF point mutation (V600E), exon 15 has to be amplified. Generally, 200 ng of template (cDNA or DNA) are added to a mix containing 200 nM of each primers, 200 μM of dNTPs, 1.5-2.5 mM $MgCl_2$ and 0.25-1.25 U Taq Polymerase. Possible primers for V600E detection are reported in Table **4** [1, 20-24]. Amplification products are then separated on an agarose gel (the percentage of the gel depends upon product size) and are visualized by ethidium

bromide. The presence of the mutation needs to be verified by DHPLC and/or direct sequencing.

**Table 4:** Primers for BRAF V600E detection [1, 20-24]

| | Primer sequences | Template | T (C°) |
|---|---|---|---|
| Set 1 | F:5'TCATAATGCTTGCTCTGATAGGA3'<br>R:5'GGCCAAAAATTTAATCAGTGGA3' | cDNA | 52.5 |
| Set 2 | F:5'GCCAAGTCAATCATCCACAG3'<br>R:5'CATCTGACTGAAAGCTGTATGGA3' | cDNA | 57 |
| Set 3 | F:5'AAACTCTTCATAATGCTTGCTCTG3'<br>R:5'GGCCAAAAATTTAATCAGTGGA-3' | DNA | Not reported |
| Set 4 | F:5'CATTGCACGACAGACTGCAC3'<br>R:5'TCTGACTGAAAGCTGTATGG3' | cDNA | 60 |

2) <u>Allele-Specific Oligonucelotides (ASO) PCR</u>: In this technique, one of the primers is designed for the polymorphic area, with the mutations located at (or near) its 3'-end. The idea is that, under stringent conditions, a mismatched primer will not initiate replication, whereas a matched primer will. The appearance of an amplification product indicates the presence of the point mutations. For BRAF V600E detection, primers are as follows: V600E F: 5'-GTGATTT-TGGTCTAGCTACAGA-3', BRAF WT F: 5'-GTGATTTTGGTCT-AGCTACAGT-3', BRAF R: 5'-TGCATTCTGATGACTTCTGG-3'. PCR is carried out with 0.5 μM each primer, 1.5 mM $MgCl_2$ and approximately 500 ng of template. Annealing temperature is 58°C for 30 sec for 35 cycles.

3) <u>Real Time PCR</u>: Real time PCR analysis can be, also, applied for BRAF point mutations [8]. Amplification is performed using 5-50 ng of template, 40 pmol of each primer, 2 pmol of each probe in a real

time PCR Master mix, for 40 cycles at 54°C. Primer and probe sequences are as follows: F: 5'-TCATAATGCTTGCTCTGATAGGA-3', R: 5'-GGCCAAAAATTTA-ATCAGTGGA-3', probe 1: 5'-AGCTACAGTGAAATCTCGATGGAG-FL-3', probe 2: 5'-LCRed705-GGTCCCATCAGTTTGAACAGTTGT-CTGGA-P-3'. After, a post amplification fluorescence melting curve is performed by gradual heating at a rate of 0.1°C/sec from 45°C to 95°C. Different DNA sequences give different melting profiles with a melting peak temperature of 59°C for the V600E and 63°C for the wild type.

4)  Colorimetric Mutector Assay (TrimGen, Sparks, MD): In this method, a detection primer is designed to block primer extension when the target base is not mutated (wild type). As a result, labelled nucleotides are not incorporated and no colorimetric reaction occurs [25].

5)  Dual Priming Oligo-nucleotide (DPO) PCR: The DPO (dual priming oligonucleotide) is composed of three regions, a longer 5'-segment, a shorter 3'-segment and a poly(I) linker that bridges these two segments. The linker assumes a bubble-like structure which itself is not involved in priming. The longer 5'-segment initiates stable priming, and the short 3'-segment determines target specific extension. This DPO-based system is a fundamental tool for blocking extension of non-specifically primed templates, and thereby generates consistently high PCR specificity even under less than optimal PCR conditions. Using this technique it is possible to lower the risk of mismatched priming which cannot be avoided in the commonly used primer systems. This type of analysis can also be used for RAS mutation detection.

6)  Mutant Enrichment with 3'-Modified Oligonucleotide (MEMO): MEMO is based on the use of a 3'-modified oligo primer that blocks

extension of the normal allele but enables extension of the mutated allele. In detail, the 3'-end of a primer, perfectly matching the wild-type sequence and encompassing the target mutation site, is modified with extension-inhibiting compounds. The overlapping generic primer neighbours the mutation site and is in competition with the blocking primer for DNA binding. For normal sequences, the DNA binding of the blocking primer, which has a higher Tm and a higher concentration, dominates that of the generic primer. For mutant sequences, the mismatches between the blocking primer and the target sequence result in reduced affinity and increases the chance for annealing of overlapping generic primers, allowing the enrichment of mutant sequences. After amplification, mutant alleles are detected by standard downstream methods such as Sanger or pyrosequencing [26, 27].

7) Allele-specific Real Time PCR [28]: This method is highly sensitive and capable of detecting BRAFV600E mutation at concentrations approaching the theoretical limit for a given BRAFV600E DNA input. The detection level is approximately 1:100,000 cells. In this method, primer and probes are designed to bind at the mutation site, acting as a primer for allele-specific extension. Both wild type and mutant primer-probes contain an additional sequence change that destabilizes primer binding, avoiding non -specific amplification. The thermal cycle profile is composed by Taq activation followed by 50 cycles of annealing at 58°C for 60 sec and melting at 95°C for 15 sec (transition rate of 3 C7s). Examples of the primers and probes are listed in Table **5**.

8) Real-time quantitative Gap Ligase Chain Reaction (GLCR) [29]: In this method, two adjacent oligonucleotide primers hybridizing to a single strand of DNA ligate only if there is an exact match to the

target sequence. No ligation occur in case of a mismatch. Exponential increase of this reaction is possible by adding complementary primers to the perfect-match cDNA strand. After Taq activation, the reaction conditions are 40 cycles at 50°C for 30 sec and 96°C for 30 sec.

**Table 5:** Primers and probe for allele specific real time PCR (28)

| Primer/probe | Nucleotide sequence and modifications (5'-3') |
|---|---|
| Wild-type BRAF Forward | GATTTTGGTCATGCTACAGT |
| Complementary strand wild-type BRAF probe | CACTCCATCGAGATTTCACTG |
| BRAF V600E-mutant allele specific Forward | GATTTTGGTCATGCTACAGA |
| Complementary strand BRAF V600E probe | CACTCCATCGAGATTTCTCTG |
| Common reverse primer | AATTCTTACCATCCACAAAA |

## Final Suggestions

The techniques proposed are all highly specific and reproducible. Which technique to select depends on sample quality and quantity and if DNA or cDNA is being used. In the presence of small quantities of starting material, classical PCR is not a good choice. It requires a test such as DHPLC or direct sequencing. The standard method for sequencing (Sanger) is high reliable but it is not sensitive enough to detect the mutation when present at low frequency. Under these conditions, real-time PCR, ASO-PCR and, even more so, DPO or MEMO [26] represent the best options. For these techniques, the use of a positive sample as a control is recommended. Real-time PCR with melting curve with classical sequence-specific probes does not allow reliable detection of mutant to wild type concentrations with ratios of much less than 1:4-1:10. Allele-specific PCR has a detection limit of 1:100 and DHPLC or direct sequencing even less than 1:4. The real time quantitative Gap ligase chain reaction can detect BRAF mutation up to a concentration level of 1/1000 copies.

## METHODS FOR THE STUDY OF PAX8/PPARγ REARRANGEMENTS

1) <u>Real-time PCR</u>: To perform this analysis [8], 5-50 ng of cDNA are amplified in a final volume of 50 μl using 40 pmol of specific primers, 2 pmol of probes for 40 cycles at 72°C. Oligonuclotide sequences are: PAX8 (exon7)-F: 5'-AACCTCTCGACTCACCAGACCTA-3', PAX8 (exon9)-F: 5'-CGGACAGGGCAGCTATGC-3', PPARγ-R: 5'-GTTGGTGGGCCAGAATGG-3', PPARγ Probe 5'-6FAM-CATGGTTGACACAGAGAT-MGBNFQ-3'.

2) <u>Nested PCR [1, 30]</u>: For the first amplifications, two forward primers designed for exon 4 and exon 5 of PAX8 gene are used (PAX8/exon4 F: 5'-CAGAACCCTACCATGTTTGCC-3', PAX8/exon5 F: 5'-GCCACCAAGTCCCTGAGTCC-3') with a PPARγ/exon1 reverse primer (5'-CAAAGGAGTGGGAGTGGTCT-3'). In the nested PCR, 1 μl of the first round is used as template with primers forward designed for exons 7 and 8 of the PAX8 gene (PAX8/exon7 F: 5'-GCATTGACTCACAGAGCAGCA-3', PAX8/exon8 F(1): 5'-GCTC-AACAGCACCCTGGA-3', PAX8/exon7 F(2): 5'-GCAACCTCCTC-GACTCACCAG-3') and primer reverse (?reverse primers) for PPARγ/exon1 (5'-CATTACGGAGAGATCCACGG-3'). Amplification mix contains 1.5 mM MgCl₂, 10 pmol of each primers and the thermal cycling conditions are 94° C for 10 min, followed by 35 cycles of 95° C for 10 sec, annealing 55° C for 10 sec, 72° C for 1 min and a final extension of 10 min at 72° C. Other different primers and conditions for nested PCR are reported by Hibi *et al.* [31].

3) <u>PCR</u>: In the presence of highly degraded RNA, it is preferable to amplify short sequences. For that, a standard PCR can be performed using forward primers for PAX8 exons 7, 8 and 9 and a common reverse primer designed for exon 1 of PPARγ gene (Table **6**) in order

to take in account the several RNA transcripts for PAX8-PPARγ chimeric protein [32].

**Table 6:** Primers for PAX8-PPARγ detection [29]

| Pax8 exon7 | 5'-AACCTCTCGACTCACCAGAC-3' |
|---|---|
| Pax8 exon 8 | 5'-CCCTTCAATGCCTTTCCCC-3' |
| Pax8 exon9 | 5'-CTATGCCTCCTCTGCCATC-3' |
| PPARγ exon 1 | 5'-AGAATGGCATCTCTGTGTCAAC-3' |

For PCR, cDNA is amplified in a final volume of 30-50 μl containing 200 nM of each primer, 200 μM of dNTPs, 1.5-2.5 mM MgCl$_2$ and 0.25-1.25 U Taq Polymerase. Annealing temperature is 60°C and thermal cycle is carried out for 35 repetitions. After, the PCR products (approximately 67-69 bp) are resolved by electrophoresis in a 2-2.5% agarose gel, visualized by ethidium bromide and directly sequenced to verify the presence of the chimeric protein.

**Final Suggestions**

The techniques proposed are reproducible and effective to detect the presence of the rearrangements. In case of low quantities of starting material, real-time PCR is preferable, whereas in case of highly degraded RNA, standard PCR is the goal standard. Whatever methods are used, the addition of a positive control is strongly recommended.

**METHODS FOR THE STUDY OF NTRK1 REARRANGEMENTS**

1) Nested PCR: TRK rearrangement (NTRK1 and TPM3, see chapter 4) can be searched with primary and nested PCR amplification followed by 1.2% agarose gel electrophoresis. Generally, 500 ng of cDNA are amplified with specific primers: forward primer is designed for the 5' region of TMP3 and reverse primer for the TK domain of NTRK-1. For nested PCR, 1:10 dilution of the first round PRC is used. Thermal

cycling conditions for both amplifications are 94° C for 5 min followed by 35 cycles at 94° C for 30 sec, 60° C for 30 sec, 72° C for 30 sec and a final extension at 72° C for 10 min [1, 12]. Primer sequences are as follows: TRK F: 5'-TGAGCAGATTAGA-CTGATGG-3', TRK R: 5'-GGAAGAGGCAGGCAAAGAC-3', TRK nested F: 5'-GCTGCCGAAGAAAAGTACTC-3', TRK nested R: 5'-TTTCGTCCTTCTTCTCCACC-3'.

2)  Standard PCR: For the study of TRK3 (NTRK1 and TGF, see chapter 4) a method has been proposed on cultured fibroblast [33]. With this method, full-length TRK3 cDNA is amplified by using primers F 5'-AACATCCTGGAGTCCACCAT-3' and R 5'-TTTTTTTTCAAGGGATAATAAA-3'. Reactions are performed in a final volume of 100 µl containing 1.5 mM $MgCl_2$, 200 µM dNTPs, 20 pM each primer and 2 U of enzyme. After a 2 min of denaturation at 92°C, 30 cycles of PCR are carried out (94°C for 20 s, 52°C for 20 s, 72°C for 100 s) and are, then, followed by a final extension at 72°C for 5 min. PCR product are electrophoresed on a 2% agarose gel and visualized by ethidium bromide staining. This method, however, has never been applied on thyroid cells or FNA. Instead, other standard PCR methods have been developed to study TRK and TRK2 (rearrangements with TPM3 and TPR, respectively. See chapter 4). For TRK [34], the cDNA fragments are amplified for 30 cycles using an annealing temperature of 56°C, 1.5 mM $MgCl_2$ and 10 µM of the following primers: TRK F: 5'-CGGGACATCGTGCTCAAGTG-3' and TRK R: 5'-AGCTTGCCGTAGGTGAAGAT-3'.

For TRK2 rearrangement [35], the cDNA fragments are amplified in a mixture containing 200 µM dNTPs, 2 mM $MgCl_2$, 2.5 U Taq Polymerase and 45 pM of the following primers: TPR F: 5'-TAATATGGAAGTCCAAGTT-3' and NTRK1

R: 5'-CACTTGAGCACGATGTC-3'. Thermal cycling conditions are: initial denaturation at 94°C for 3 min, 30 cycles of PCR (94°C for 30 sec, 56°C for 30 sec and 72°C for 90 sec) followed by a final extension of 7-10 min at 72°C.

## OUR EXPERIENCE AND THAT OF OTHERS

Many studies have demonstrated the feasibility of mutation detection in FNA samples from thyroid nodules and their contribution in improving the diagnostic accuracy of FNAC. The identification of BRAF mutations in cytological material was first reported by Cohen [36] with good results, and this was subsequently confirmed by other authors [23, 37, 38]. However, BRAF mutations account for no more than 30-40% of papillary thyroid carcinomas and thus does not cover the entire spectrum of thyroid malignancies. Other authors have searched for a panel of oncogene mutations, including BRAF, RET/PTC and TRK [12, 15, 20]. All of these authors have concluded that the identification of BRAF or RET/PTC refines the diagnosis of papillary thyroid cancer, especially in FNAC with indeterminate cytology. However, the ideal tool would be able to identify all oncogenes involved in thyroid tumorigenesis. This approach has been developed by Nikiforov [8] and by our laboratory [1]. Nikiforov *et al.* prospectively tested FNA samples of thyroid nodules for BRAF, RAS, RET/PTC and PAX8/PPRγ. At final histology, 97% of 31 thyroid cancers were associated with a mutation of either BRAF, RAS, RET/PTC or PAX8/PPARγ, demonstrating that the presence of any of these mutations is a strong indicator of thyroid cancer. In particular, the presence of BRAF mutation and RET/PTC rearrangement had a 100% positive predictive value for papillary carcinoma, while the presence of RAS mutation conferred an 87.5% probability of malignancy. The authors concluded that the combination of cytology and molecular testing improves diagnostic accuracy and helps in refining patient management and in reducing surgical costs and morbidity.

The study by Cantara *et al.* [1] analyzed the presence of BRAF, RAS, RET/PTC, TRK, and PAX8/PPARγ mutations in 235 FNAC and the corresponding tumoral tissues taken at surgery. Mutations were found in 28.5% of the cytological samples and were always confirmed in the tissue sample. The presence of mutations at cytology was associated with cancer 91.1% of the time and with follicular adenoma 8.9% of the time, but never with hyperplastic nodules. Similarly to the results of Nikiforov, BRAF or RET/PTC mutations were always associated with cancer, while RAS mutations were mainly associated with cancer (74%) but also with follicular adenoma (26%). The diagnostic performance of the molecular analysis was superior to that of traditional cytology, with better sensitivity and specificity, and the combination of the two techniques further contributed to improve the total accuracy (95.7%), compared to molecular analysis (92.8%) or traditional cytology (83.0%) alone. Overall, the association of oncogene analysis and traditional cytology increases the diagnostic detection of thyroid cancer and may help to choose the best therapeutic approach. A recent study [3], analyzed 1056 consecutive thyroid FNA samples with indeterminate cytology, and found adequate material for molecular analysis in 967 (92%). In total they found 87 mutations (8.9%): 19 BRAF, 62 RAS, 1 RET/PTC and 5 PAX8/PPARγ. Of these 87 nodules, 83 contained cancer at histology confirming that molecular analysis for a panel of mutations ameliorates the clinical management of patients with indeterminate cytology.

At present, the use of molecular biology for the evaluation of genetic alterations in FNAC samples has some limitations. These include issues related to the technique (RNA recovery and subjective interpretation of the results) and to the operator (time-consuming procedures and need of specialized laboratories). We hope that the suggestions provided in this chapter will help many laboratories overcome these limitations.

## WHAT LIES AHEAD?

Based on the above observations, the future in the field of thyroid cancer diagnosis may bring the development and validation of a single platform for the simultaneous analysis of all the genetic alterations involved in thyroid cancer on cytological material obtained from fine-needle aspiration. Such an approach will allow, in a single experiment, the analysis of all the genetic markers of malignancy thus optimizing the cost-benefit ratio, the time required for the experiments and the reliability of the results. Recently, Chudova *et al.* [39] developed a molecular test using more than 247186 transcripts that identifies benign thyroid nodules from fine-needle aspirates, obtaining a negative predictive value and specificity of 96 and 84%, respectively. The authors searched for a generic panel of gene expression to identify benign nodules instead of searching for established markers of malignancy, but their experience demonstrated that an array approach is possible.

## CONFLICT OF INTEREST

The author confirms that she has no conflicts of interest.

## ACKNOWLEDGEMENTS

Declared none.

## REFERENCES

[1]    Cantara S, Capezzone M, Marchisotta S, Capuano S, Busonero G, Toti P, Di Santo A, Caruso G, Carli AF, Brilli L, Montanaro A, Pacini F. Impact of proto-oncogene mutation detection in cytological specimens from thyroid nodules improves the diagnostic accuracy of cytology. J Clin Endocrinol Metab. 2010, 95:1365-9.

[2]    Sambrook and Russell. Molecular Cloning: A Laboratory Manual (3rd ed.). 2001, Cold Spring Harbor Laboratory Press.

[3]    Nikiforov YE, Ohori NP, Hodak SP, Carty SE, LeBeau SO, Ferris RL, Yip L, Seethala RR, Tublin ME, Stang MT, Coyne C, Johnson JT, Stewart AF, Nikiforova MN.

Impact of mutational testing on the diagnosis and management of patients with cytologically indeterminate thyroid nodules: a prospective analysis of 1056 FNA samples. J Clin Endocrinol Metab. 2011, 96:3390-7.

[4]     Vasko V, Ferrand M, Di Cristofaro J, Carayon P, Henry JF, de Micco C. Specific pattern of RAS oncogene mutations in follicular thyroid tumors. JCEM 2003, 88:2745-52.

[5]     Volante M, Rapa I, Gandhi M, Bussolati G, Giachino D, Papotti M, Nikiforov YE. RAS mutations are the predominant molecular alteration in poorly differentiated thyroid carcinomas and bear prognostic impact. JCEM 2009, 94: 4735-41.

[6]     Cantara S, Capuano S, Formichi C, Pisu M, Capezzone M, Pacini F. Lack of germline A339V mutation in thyroid transcription factor-1 (TITF-1/NKX2.1) gene in familial papillary thyroid cancer. Thyroid Res. 2010, 3:4.

[7]     Nikiforova MN, Lynch RA, Biddinger PW, Alexander EK, Dorn GW 2nd, Tallini G, Kroll TG, Nikiforov YE. RAS point mutations and PAX8-PPAR gamma rearrangement in thyroid tumors: evidence for distinct molecular pathways in thyroid follicular carcinoma. JCEM 2003, 88:2318-26.

[8]     Nikiforov YE, Steward DL, Robinson-Smith TM, Haugen BR, Klopper JP, Zhu Z, Fagin JA, Falciglia M, Weber K, Nikiforova MN. Molecular testing for mutations in improving the fine-needle aspiration diagnosis of thyroid nodules. J Clin Endocrinol Metab. 2009, 94:2092-8.

[9]     Wittwer CT, Herrmann MG, Moss AA, Rasmussen RP. Continuous fluorescence monitoring of rapid cycle DNA amplification. Biotechniques 1992, 22:130-131, 134-138.

[10]    Ibrahem S, Seth R, O'Sullivan B, Fadhil W, Taniere P, Ilyas M. Comparative analysis of pyrosequencing and QMC-PCR in conjunction with high resolution melting for KRAS/BRAF mutation detection. Int J Exp Pathol. 2010, 91:500-5.

[11]    Kramer D, Thunnissen FB, Gallegos-Ruiz MI, Smit EF, Postmus PE, Meijer CJ, Snijders PJ, Heideman DA. A fast, sensitive and accurate high resolution melting (HRM) technology-based assay to screen for common K-ras mutations. Cell Oncol 2009, 31:161-7.

[12]    Sapio MR, Posca D, Raggioli A, Guerra A, Marotta V, Deandrea M, Motta M, Limone PP, Troncone G, Caleo A, Rossi G, Fenzi G, Vitale M. Detection of RET/PTC, TRK and BRAF mutations in preoperative diagnosis of thyroid nodules with indeterminate cytological findings. Clin Endocrinol (Oxf). 2007, 66:678-83.

[13]    Elisei R, Romei C, Vorontsova T, Cosci B, Veremeychik V, Kuchinskaya E, Basolo F, Demidchik EP, Miccoli P, Pinchera A, Pacini F. RET/PTC rearrangements in thyroid nodules: studies in irradiated and not irradiated, malignant and benign thyroid lesions in children and adults. J Clin Endocrinol Metab. 2001, 86:3211-6.

[14]    Fugazzola L, Pilotti S, Pinchera A, Vorontsova TV, Mondellini P, Bongarzone I, Greco A, Astakhova L, Butti MG, Demidchik EP, Pacini F, Pienotti M. Oncogenic rearrangements of the RET proto-oncogene in papillary thyroid carcinomas from children exposed to the Chernobyl nuclear accident. Cancer Res. 1995, 55:5617-20.

[15]    Pizzolanti G, Russo L, Richiusa P, Bronte V, Nuara RB, Rodolico V, Amato MC, Smeraldi L, Sisto PS, Nucera M, Bommarito A, Citarrella R, Lo Coco R, Cabibi D, Lo Coco A, Frasca F, Gulotta G, Latteri MA, Modica G, Galluzzo A, Giordano C. Fine-needle aspiration molecular analysis for the diagnosis of papillary thyroid carcinoma through BRAF V600E mutation and RET/PTC rearrangement. Thyroid. 2007, 17:1109-15.

[16]    Learoyd DL, Messina M, Zedenius J, Guinea AI, Delbridge LW, Robinson BG. RET/PTC and RET tyrosine kinase expression in adult papillary thyroid carcinomas. JCEM 1998, 83:3631-5.

[17]    Zhu Z, Ciampi R, Nikiforova MN, Gandhi M, Nififorov Y. Prevalence of RET/PTC rearrangements in thyroid papillary carcinomas: effects of the detection methods and genetic heterogeneity. JCEM 2006, 91:3603-3610.

[18]    Rhoden KJ, Unger K, Salvatore G, Yilmaz Y, Vovk V, Chiappetta G, Qumsiyeh MB, Rothstein JL, Fusco A, Santoro M, Zitzelsberger H, Tallini G. RET/papillary thyroid cancer rearrangement in nonneoplastic thyrocytes: follicular cells of Hashimoto's thyroiditis share low-level recombination events with a subset of papillary carcinoma. JCEM 2006, 91:2414-23.

[19]    Rhoden KJ, Johnson C, Brandao G, Howe JG, Smith BR, Tallini G. Real-time quantitative RT-PCR identifies distinct c-RET, RET/PTC1 and RET/PTC3 expression patterns in papillary thyroid carcinoma. Lab Invest 2004, 84:1557-70.

[20]    Domingues R, Mendonça E, Sobrinho L, Bugalho MJ. Searching for RET/PTC rearrangements and BRAF V599E mutation in thyroid aspirates might contribute to establish a preoperative diagnosis of papillary thyroid carcinoma. Cytopathology. 2005, 16:27-31.

[21]    Kimura ET, Nikiforova MN, Zhu Z, Knauf JA, Nikiforov YE, Fagin JA. High prevalence of BRAF mutations in thyroid cancer: genetic evidence for constitutive activation of the RET/PTC-RAS-BRAF signaling pathway in papillary thyroid carcinoma. Cancer Res. 2003, 63:1454-7.

[22]    Puxeddu E, Moretti S, Elisei R, Romei C, Pascucci R, Martinelli M, Marino C, Avenia N, Rossi ED, Fadda G, Cavaliere A, Ribacchi R, Falorni A, Pontecorvi A, Pacini F, Pinchera A, Santeusanio F. BRAF(V599E) mutation is the leading genetic event in adult sporadic papillary thyroid carcinomas. JCEM 2004, 89:2414-2420.

[23]    Xing M, Tufano RP, Tufaro AP, Basaria S, Ewertz M, Rosenbaum E, Byrne PJ, Wang J, Sidransky D, Ladenson PW. Detection of BRAF mutation on fine needle aspiration biopsy specimens: a new diagnostic tool for papillary thyroid cancer. J Clin Endocrinol Metab. 2004, 89:2867-72.

[24]    Salvatore G, Giannini R, Faviana P, Caleo A, Migliaccio I, Fagin JA, Nikiforov YE, Troncone G, Palombini L, Basolo F, Santoro M. Analysis of BRAF point mutation and RET/PTC rearrangement refines the fine-needle aspiration diagnosis of papillary thyroid carcinoma. JCEM 2004, 89:5175-5180.

[25]    Cohen Y, Rosenbaum E, Clark DP, Geiger MA, Umbricht CB, Tufano RP, Sidransky D, Westra WH. Mutational analysis of BRAF in fine needle aspiration biopsies of the thyroid. A potential application for the preoperative assessment of thyroid nodules. Clin Cancer Res 2004, 10:2761-2765.

[26]    Lee ST, Kim SW, Ki CS, Jang JH, Shin JH, Oh YL, Kim JW, Chung JH. Clinical Implication of Highly Sensitive Detection of the BRAF V600E Mutation in Fine-Needle Aspirations of Thyroid Nodules: A Comparative Analysis of Three Molecular Assays in 4585 Consecutive Cases in a BRAF V600E Mutation-Prevalent Area. JCEM April, 2012 [Epub ahead of print].

[27]    Lee ST, Kim JY, Kown MJ, Kim SW, Chung JH, Ahn MJ, Oh YL, Kim JW, Ki CS. Mutant enrichment with 3'-modified oligonucleotides: a pratical PCR method for detecting trace mutant DNAs. J Mol Diagn 2011, 13:657-668.

[28]    Candric KW, Milosevic D, Rosenberg AM, Erickson LA, McIver B, Grebe SKG. Mutant BRAF T1799A can be detected in the blood of papillary thyroid carcinoma patients and correlates with disease status. JCEM 2009, 94:5001-5009.

[29]    Chuang TC, Chuang AYC, Poeta L, Koch WM, Califano JA, Tufano RP. Detectable BRAF mutation in serum DNA samples from patients with papillary thyroid carcinoma. Head and neck 2010, 32:229-34.

[30]    Marques AR, Espadinha C, Catarino AL, Moniz S, Pereira T, Sobrinho LG, Leite V. Expression of PAX8-PPAR gamma 1 rearrangements in both follicular thyroid carcinomas and adenomas. JCEM 2002, 87:3947-3952.

[31]    Hibi Y, Nagaya T, Kambe F, Imai T, Funahashi H, Nakao A, Seo H. Is thyroid follicular cancer in Japanese caused by a specific t(2; 3)(q13; p25) translocation generating Pax8-PPAR gamma fusion mRNA? Endocr J. 2004, 51:361-6.

[32]    Nikiforova MN, Biddinger PW, Caudill CM, Kroll TG, Nikiforov YE. Pax8-PPARgamma rearrangement in thyroid tumors. RT-PCR and immunohistochemical analyses. The American J of Surg Pathol 2002, 26:1016-1023.

[33]    Greco A, Mariani C, Miranda C, Lupas A, Pagliardini S, Pomati M, Pierotti MA. The DNA rearrangement that generates the TRK-T3 oncogene involves a novel gene on chromosome 3 whose product has a potential coiled-coil domain. Mol Cell Biol. 1995, 15:6118-27.

[34]    Bongarzone I, Fugazzola L, Vigneri P, Mariani L, Mondellini P, Pacini F, Basolo F, Pinchera A, Pilotti S, Pierotti MA. Age-related activation of the tyrosine kinase receptor protooncogenes RET and NTRK1 in papillary thyroid carcinoma. JCEM 1996, 81:2006-9.

[35]    Greco A, Miranda C, Pagliardini S, Fusetti L, Bongarzone I, Pierotti MA. Chromosome 1 rearrangements involving the genes TPR and NTRK1 produce structurally different thyroid-specific TRK oncogenes. Genes, chromosomes and Cancer 1997, 19:112-123.

[36]    Cohen Y, Rosenbaum E, Begum S, Goldenberg D, Esche C, Lavie O, Sidransky D, Westra WH. Exon 15 BRAF mutations are uncommon in melanomas arising in nonsun-exposed sites. Clin Cancer Res. 2004, 10:3444-7.

[37]    Chung KW, Yang SK, Lee GK, Kim EY, Kwon S, Lee SH, Park do J, Lee HS, Cho BY, Lee ES, Kim SW. Detection of BRAFV600E mutation on fine needle aspiration specimens of thyroid nodule refines cyto-pathology diagnosis, especially in BRAF600E mutation-prevalent area. Clin Endocrinol (Oxf). 2006, 65:660-6.

[38]    Marchetti I, Lessi F, Mazzanti CM, Bertacca G, Elisei R, Coscio GD, Pinchera A, Bevilacqua G. A morpho-molecular diagnosis of papillary thyroid carcinoma: BRAF V600E detection as an important tool in preoperative evaluation of fine-needle aspirates. Thyroid. 2009, 19:837-42.

[39]    Chudova D, Wilde JI, Wang ET, Wang H, Rabbee N, Egidio CM, Reynolds J, Tom E, Pagan M, Rigl CT, Friedman L, Wang CC, Lanman RB, Zeiger M, Kebebew E, Rosai J, Fellegara G, LiVolsi VA, Kennedy GC. Molecular classification of thyroid nodules using high-dimensionality genomic data. J Clin Endocrinol Metab. 2010, 95:5296-304.

# CHAPTER 5

# Familial Non-Medullary Thyroid Cancer

Stefania Marchisotta[*]

*Section of Endocrinology & Metabolism, Department of Medical, Surgical and Neurological Sciences University of Siena, Siena, Italy*

**Abstract:** Familial non-medullary thyroid cancer is a clear clinical distinct entity characterized by multifocality and a more severe phenotype and is defined as the presence of two or more first-degree relatives affected by differentiated thyroid cancer of follicular origin. In some cases, the disease is associated with rare hereditary syndromes such as Carney complex, Werner syndromes, FAP and Cowden syndromes. However, in the majority of the cases, patients have thyroid cancer as the only disease manifestation. Several studies have tried to identify the genetic alteration(s) responsible for the development of FNMTC with promising results although none of the genes/loci identified accounts for the majority of cases of FNMTC and cannot be generalized to the larger at-risk population.

**Keywords:** FNMTC, Cowden disease, Werner syndrome, Carney complex, genetic loci.

## DEFINITION AND INCIDENCE

Familial non-medullary thyroid cancer (FNMTC) is defined as the diagnosis of two or more first- degree relatives affected by differentiated thyroid cancer of follicular cell origin [1], as opposed to medullary thyroid cancer without germline RET proto-oncogene mutations, in which the familial form is defined as the

*Address correspondence to Stefania Marchisotta:** Section of Endocrinology & Metabolism, Department of Internal Medicine, Endocrinology & Metabolism and Biochemistry, University of Siena, Siena, Italy; E-mail: stefaniamarchisotta@libero.it

Silvia Cantara (Ed)

presence of four or more affected family members [2]. The prevalence of FNMTC is approximately 6% among patients with differentiated thyroid cancer [3]. However, the real incidence is, probably, underestimated as differentiated thyroid cancer often remains occult or presents an indolent course [4]. It is difficult to demonstrate the real existence of inherited FNMTC, and to know whether it is related to some peculiar features of the thyroid gland. First, thyroid cancer is frequently found within uni- or multinodular goiter that "*per se*" has been recognized as a familial disease [5]. In these cases, thyroid cancer may occur from somatic mutations in the background of a long-standing familial goiter. Second, the diagnosis of thyroid cancer has markedly increased since the introduction of neck ultrasound in clinical practice [6]. Some cohort-based studies [3, 7-9] have shown that the risk of developing non medullary thyroid cancer (NMTC) is significantly greater (between 3 and 9 fold) in first-degree relatives of subjects with NMTC corroborating the existence of the familial form of the disease. However, although thyroid cancer shows a highest heritability among solid tumors, genome wide association studies (GWAS) conducted on populations have detected only few loci where SNPs reached genome-wide significance and typically only a single locus was found in each pedigree raging ("raging" does not make sense; not sure what is meant here) a quite low LOD score [10-12] (see below paragraph "Genetics of FNMTC").

## ASSOCIATION WITH OTHER SYNDROMES

Several rare hereditary syndromes caused by germline mutations of known tumor suppressor genes are associated with the occurrence of differentiated thyroid cancer, mainly of the papillary histotype (PTC). Familial Adenomatous Poliposis Syndrome (FAP) has been associated with the occurrence of NMTC [13-15]. FAP is an autosomal dominant disease caused by inactivating mutations of the APC tumor suppressor gene located on chromosome 5q21. It is characterized by the development of multiple adenomatous polyps with malignant potential lining the mucosa of the gastrointestinal tract, particularly the colon. In this syndrome, PTC occurs with a frequency of about 10 times higher than expected for sporadic PTC and has an unusual cribriform pathology [14]. Later, NMTC was described with a greater frequency than expected in the Gardner's Syndrome, a variant of FAP characterized by the presence of multiple polyps in the colon together with tumors outside the colon [16].

A relationship between Cowden disease (familial hamartoma syndrome) and thyroid cancer has been also described [17]. Cowden syndrome is characterized by hamartomatous neoplasms of the skin and mucosa, gastro-intestinal tract, bones, central nervous system, eyes, and genitourinary tract. Skin is involved in 90-100% of cases, and the thyroid is involved in 66% of cases [18]. Both thyroid benign neoplasm and follicular cancer may occur. In approximately 80% of the cases, the syndrome is caused by a mutation in the PTEN (phosphatase and tensin homolog) tumor-suppressor gene located on chromosome 10q22-23 and is inherited as an autosomal dominant trait [17].

NMTC of distinct histological types can also be a component in other heritable cancer syndromes such as the Werner Syndrome (WS) [19] and the Carney Complex (CC) [20]. The WS is a disease of the connective tissue characterized by premature aging and is often referred to as "progeria". The syndrome is caused by a mutation in the Werner gene or RecQ helicase located on chromosome 8 and is inherited as an autosomal recessive disease [19]. The CC is an autosomal dominant condition comprising myxomas of the heart and skin, hyperpigmen-tation of the skin together with thyroid cancer. Approximately 70% of the cases are caused by inactivating germline mutations in the PPRKAR1-alpha (protein kinase A regulatory subunit type 1-alpha) gene located at 17q23-q24. The remaining forms are caused by genetic changes at chromosome 2p16 [20].

## FNMTC NOT ASSOCIATED WITH OTHER SYNDROMES

Although it can be associated with the above described syndromes, most of the FNMTC patients have thyroid cancer as the only disease manifestation and not associated with a distinct phenotype.

Several studies [21-23] reported that FNMTC are usually more aggressive when compared with sporadic PTC in terms of higher incidence of multifocality and local invasion and higher rate of local recurrence. In addition, FNMTC are diagnosed at younger ages compared to sporadic forms [23]. At variance with these studies, other authors [4, 24] have reported no differences in the clinical behavior of sporadic and familial PTC. A recent work by Capezzone *et al.* [23] compared the features of patients with sporadic and familial NMTC patients and tested whether FNMTC patients with parent-child relationship exhibit an "anticipation" phenomenon (earlier age at disease onset and increased severity in successive generations) [23]. According with this study, FNMTC patients showed more frequently tumor multifocality (P=0.001) and worse final outcome (P=0.001) compared to sporadic PTC. Moreover, among FNMTC cases with parent-child relationship, an earlier age at disease presentation (P<0.001), diagnosis (P<0.001), and disease onset (P=0.04) were found in the second generation when compared with the first generations. Patients in the second generation had a higher rate of lymph node metastases at surgery and worse outcome when compared with the first generation. The authors suggested that FNMTC is a true familial disease rather than the fortuitous association of the same disease in a family.

## GENETICS OF FNMTC

So far, no candidate gene(s) has been discovered for this form of isolated familial DTC and only in a minority of cases have different susceptibility loci been identified at 1q21 [25, 26], 2q21 [12], 6q22 [26], 8q24 [27] and 8p23.1 [28], 14q31 [29] and 19p13.2 [11].

The first locus to be implicated in familial PTC was MNG1 which maps on chromosome 14q31 [29]. In this paper, the authors described a family from Montreal, Canada, with 18 members affected by multinodular goitre (MNG). Among these patients, two had an associated papillary thyroid cancer and one had follicular adenoma. The authors concluded that a very small proportion of familial NMTC (point estimate 0.001, support intervals 0-.6 under a dominant model) was attributable to MNG1 [29]. The locus was confirmed in other families [30], but no evidence of linkage was found in additional FNMTC pedigrees reinforcing the concept that only a small percentage of FNMTC can be attributed to this locus [31].

The TCO (Thyroid Carcinoma with Cell Oxyphilia) locus at 19p13.2 was first identified in a French family with oxyphilic thyroid neoplasms by linkage analysis with a whole-genome panel of microsatellite markers [11]. An autosomal dominant inheritance pattern with reduced penetrance appears likely in these pedigrees [11].

The PRN1 locus was identified by Malchoff *et al.* on chromosome 1q21 in an American kindred with papillary thyroid cancer, nodular thyroid disease, and papillary renal neoplasia [25]. To date, linkage to this locus has not been confirmed in any other independent study.

The existence of the susceptibility locus NMTC1 on chromosome 2q21 was established in a large Tasmanian family [12]. This locus has been associated with development of the follicular variant of papillary thyroid cancer and has been confirmed in another study on 80 additional FNMTC pedigrees [12]. There is also a recent study which demonstrates an interaction between the TCO and NMTC1 loci in a subset of FNMTC pedigrees, suggesting that both of them can interact to increase the risk of thyroid cancer [32]. However, it appears unlikely that an interaction between the TCO and NMTC1 loci is common among the majority of FNMTC pedigrees.

Related to the above described loci, most of the linkage studies have yielded a logarithm of the odds (LOD) scores less than 3, thus failing to identify the same loci, or have shown no linkage.

In 2009, a study by Suh and collaborators [26], demonstrated, using a SNP array-based linkage analysis, a linkage between FNMTC and loci at 1q21 and 6q22 in 38 families. In these sets of families, the LOD score was 3.3 and 3.04, respectively. The authors suggested the presence of germline mutations in heretofore-undiscovered genes at these loci responsible for the predisposition to develop the familial form of thyroid cancer.

In the same year, another group [27] performed a genome-wide linkage analysis in a large family with PTC and melanoma. The authors found that, among several peaks, the highest was at 8q24, with a maximum nonparametric linkage (NPL) score of 7.03. Linkage analysis carried out with 25 additional PTC families produced a maximum NPL score of 3.2 (P = 0.007). Fine mapping with microsatellite markers was compatible with linkage to the 8q24 locus in 10 of the 26 families. In this region the authors found three likely noncoding RNA genes one of which (AK023948) was significantly down-regulated in most PTC tumors rendering the putative noncoding RNA gene AK023948 a good candidate susceptibility gene for PTC [27].

Finally, the locus at chromosome 8p23.1-p22 was identified in a Portuguese family with 11 members affected with benign thyroid lesions and five affected with thyroid carcinomas using a genome-wide linkage analysis with a LOD score of 4.41 [28]. Linkage analysis with microsatellite markers confirmed linkage to 8q23.1-p22, and recombination events delimited the minimal region to a 7.46-Mb span. Again the authors concluded that mutations in gene(s) located at this region may be responsible for the development of FNMTC.

However, none of these genes/loci accounts for the majority of cases of FNMTC and most of these studies have been performed in only one or a few families, and cannot be generalized to the larger at-risk population. A summary of the identified loci and number of families involved is presented in Table **1**.

**Table 1:** Summary of the loci associated with FNMTC

| Locus | Year of Discovery | No. of Associated Families | Refs |
|---|---|---|---|
| 14q31 | 1997 | 1 | [29] |
| 19p13.2 | 1998 | 1 | [11] |
| 1q21 | 2000 | 1 | [25] |
|  | 2009 | 38 | [26] |
| 2q21 | 2001 | 1 | [12] |
| 8p23.1-p22 | 2008 | 1 | [28] |
| 8q24 | 2009 | 10 | [27] |
| 6q22 | 2009 | 38 | [26] |

Other studies have tried to analyze the involvement of the telomere-telomerase complex in the predisposition to develop familial thyroid cancer with dissimilar results. Capezzone *et al.* [33] reported that familial thyroid cancer patients displayed short telomeres, *hTERT* gene amplification, and increased hTERT expression in the peripheral blood compared to sporadic forms, benign thyroid diseases, healthy subjects and unaffected family members. The authors suggested that FNMTC patients are born with short telomeres and thus might reach, earlier in life, the threshold telomere length sufficient to trigger cancer development and/or progression. This was consistent with the observation that familial patients of the second generation were always diagnosed with thyroid cancer at an earlier age compared to their affected relative in the first generation. The germline nature of the shorter telomere length observed in FNMTC patients was confirmed by the same authors in a second paper [34] in which they analyzed the relative telomere length at somatic level in neoplastic and non-neoplastic tissues of 30 FNMTC patients compared to 46 sporadic PTC patients. While the telomere length (TL) was reduced in both sporadic tumours and, even more, in familial tumours, the TL of normal thyroid tissues and extra-thyroidal tissues differed in the two cohorts of patients. In familial cases, TL was similarly short in any tissue examined, while in sporadic cases normal thyroid tissues and extra-thyroidal tissues had longer telomeres compared to the primary tumour. These data confirmed that in familial patients the presence of short telomeres is a peculiar feature of all the cells of the body, likely inherited from the parents [34]. From the moment that short telomeres in the genome have been associated with chromosome instability [35], some authors demonstrated an increased presence of telomere abnormalities (such as telomere fusions and associations) and chromosome fragility in patients affected by familial papillary thyroid cancer compared to sporadic patients, healthy subjects and unaffected family members [36]. However, the association between short telomeres and FNMTC was not confirmed by another group which found no variations in the TL, *hTERT* gene amplification and hTERT expression in the peripheral blood of FNMTC compared to sporadic cases and general population [37] opening a debate on this issue.

In 2009, Ngan *et al.* [38] demonstrated the presence of a germline mutation (A339V) in thyroid transcription factor-1 (TITF-1/NKX2.1) in patients with multinodular goiter and papillary thyroid carcinoma. In this study, the alteration was identified in 20% of MNG/PTC patients which developed more advanced tumors than MNG/PTC or PTC patients without the mutation and it was dominantly inherited in two families. In contrast, a study conducted in 2010 on 63 FMTC patients both with parent-child or sibling relationships showed the absence of the A339V mutation in these families [39].

# CONCLUSIONS

In conclusion, non-medullary thyroid cancer is the most common type of thyroid cancer and its familial form is increasingly recognized as a distinct clinical entity characterized by multifocality and a more severe phenotype than its sporadic counterpart. However, the genetic background of FNMTC is still poorly understood and the causative gene(s) have not yet been identified in majority of the cases. Discovering the causative mutation(s) involved in this pathology will also provide a powerful tool for the screening of the general population in order to identify subjects at higher risk to develop FNTC.

# CONFLICT OF INTEREST

The author confirm that he has no conflicts of interest.

# ACKNOWLEDGEMENTS

Declared none.

# REFERENCES

[1]     Sippel RS, Caron NR, Clark OH. An Evidence-based Approach to Familial Nonmedullary Thyroid Cancer: Screening, Clinical Management, and Follow-up. World J of Surgery 2007, 31:924-933.

[2]     Mulligan LM, Marsh DJ, Robinson BG, Schuffenecker I, Zedenius J, Lips CJ, Gagel RF, Takai SI, Noll WW, Fink M, *et al.* Genotype-phenotype correlation in multiple endocrine neoplasia type 2: report of the International RET Mutation Consortium. J Intern Med. 1995, 238:343-6.

[3]     Frich L, Glattre E, Akslen LA. Familial occurrence of nonmedullary thyroid cancer: a population-based study of 5673 first-degree relatives of thyroid cancer patients from Norway. Cancer Epidemiol Biomarkers Prev. 2001, 10:113-7.

[4]     Loh KC. Familial nonmedullary thyroid carcinoma: a meta-review of case series. Thyroid 1997, 7:107-13.

[5]     Krohn K, Fuhrer D, Bayer Y, Eszlinger M, Brauer V, Neumann S, Paschke R. Molecular Pathogenesis of Euthyroid and Toxic Multinodular Goiter. Endocrine Reviews 2005, 26:504–524.

[6]     Davies L, Welch HG. Increasing incidence of thyroid cancer in the United States, 1973-2002. JAMA. 2006, 295:2164-7.

[7]     Goldgar DE, Easton DF, Cannon-Albright LA, Skolnick MH. Systematic Population-Based Assessment of Cancer Risk in First-Degree Relatives of Cancer Probands. JNCI J Natl Cancer Inst 1994, 86: 1600-1608.

[8]     Pal T, Vogl FD, Chappuis PO, Tsang R, Brierley J, Renard H, Sanders K, Kantemiroff T, Bagha S, Goldgar DE, Narod SA, Foulkes W. Increased Risk for Nonmedullary Thyroid Cancer in the First Degree Relatives of Prevalent Cases of Nonmedullary Thyroid Cancer: A Hospital-Based Study. JCEM 2001, 86:5307-5312.

[9]     Grossman RF, Tu SH, Duh QY, Siperstein AE, Novosolov F, Clark OH. Familial nonmedullary thyroid cancer. An emerging entity that warrants aggressive treatment. Arch Surg. 1995, 130:892-7.

[10]    Gudmundsson J, Sulem P, Gudbjartsson DF, Jonasson JG, Sigurdsson A, Bergthorsson JT, He H, Blondal T, Geller F, Jakobsdottir M, Magnusdottir DN, Matthiasdottir S, Stacey SN, Skarphedinsson OB, Helgadottir H, Li W, Nagy R, Aguillo E, Faure E, Prats E, Saez B, Martinez M, Eyjolfsson GI, Bjornsdottir US, Holm H, Kristjansson K, Frigge ML, Kristvinsson H, Gulcher JR, Jonsson T, Rafnar T, Hjartarsson H, Mayordomo JI, de la Chapelle A, Hrafnkelsson J, Thorsteinsdottir U, Kong A, Stefansson K. Common variants on 9q22.33 and 14q13.3 predispose to thyroid cancer in European populations. Nat Gen. 2009, 41:460-4.

[11]    Canzian F, Amati P, Harach HR, Kraimps JL, Lesueur F, Barbier J, Levillain P, Romeo G, Bonneau D. A gene predisposing to familial thyroid tumors with cell oxyphilia maps to chromosome 19p13.2. Am J Human Genet 1998, 63:1743-1748.

[12]    McKay JD, Lesueur F, Jonard L, Pastore A, Williamson J, Hoffman L, Burgess J, Duffield A, Papotti M, Stark M, Sobol H, Maes B, Murat A, Kääriäinen H, Bertholon-Grégoire M, Zini M, Rossing MA, Toubert ME, Bonichon F, Cavarec M, Bernard AM, Boneu A, Leprat F, Haas O, Lasset C, Schlumberger M, Canzian F, Goldgar DE, Romeo G. Localization of a susceptibility gene for familial nonmedullary thyroid carcinoma to chromosome 2q21. Am J Hum Genet 2001, 69:440-446.

[13]    Perrier ND, van Heerden JA, Goellner JR, Williams ED, Gharib H, Marchesa P, Church JM, Fazio VW, Larson DR. Thyroid cancer in patients with familial adenomatous polyposis. World J Surg. 1998, 22:738-42.

[14]    Hizawa K, Iida M, Yao T, Aoyagi K, Oohata Y, Mibu R, Yamasaki K, Hirata T, Fujishima M. Association between thyroid cancer of cribriform variant and familial adenomatous polyposis. J Clin Pathol. 1996, 49:611–613.

[15]    Lee S, Hong SW, Shin SJ, Kim YM, Rhee Y, Jeon BI, Moon WC, Oh MR, Lim SK. Papillary thyroid carcinoma associated with familial adenomatous polyposis: molecular analysis of pathogenesis in a family and review of the literature. Endocr J. 2004, 51:317-23.

[16] Hizawa K, Iida M, Aoyagi K, Yao T, Fujishima M. Thyroid neoplasia and familial adenomatous polyposis/Gardner's syndrome. J Gastroenterol. 1997, 32:196-9.

[17] Liaw D, Marsh DJ, Li J, Dahia PLM, Wang SI, Zheng Z, Bose S, Call KM, Tsou HC, Peacocke M, Eng C, Parsons R Germline mutations of the PTEN gene in Cowden disease, an inherited breast and thyroid cancer syndrome. Nat Genet 1997, 16: 64-67.

[18] Mallory SB. Cowden syndrome (multiple hamartoma syndrome). Dermatol Clin. 1995, 13:27-31.

[19] Goto M, Miller RW, Ishikawa Y, Sugano H. Excess of rare cancers in (adult progeria). Cancer Epidemiol Biomarkers Prev 1996, 5:239-246.

[20] Stratakis CA, Courcoutsakies NA, Abati A, Filie A, Doppman JL, Carney A, Shawker T. Thyroid gland abnormalities in patients with the syndrome of spotty skin pigmentation, myxomas, endocrine overactivity, and schwannomas (Carney Complex). JCEM 1997, 82:2037–43.

[21] Triponez F, Wong M, Sturgeon C, Caron N, Ginzinger DG, Segal MR, Kebebew E, Duh QY & Clark OH. Does familial non-medullary thyroid cancer adversely affect survival? World Journal of Surgery 2006, 30:787–793.

[22] Alsanea O, Wada N, Ain K, Wong M, Taylor K, Ituarte PH, Treseler PA, Weier HU, Freimer N, Siperstein AE *et al.* Is familial non-medullary thyroid carcinoma more aggressive than sporadic thyroid cancer? A multicenter series. Surgery 2000, 128:1043–1051.

[23] Capezzone M, Marchisotta S, Cantara S, Busonero G, Brilli L, Pazaitou-Panayiotou K. Familial non-medullary thyroid carcinoma displays the features of clinical anticipation suggestive of a distinct biological entity. Endocrine-Related Cancer 2008,15:1075–1081.

[24] Maxwell EL, Hall FT, Freeman JL. Familial non- medullary thyroid cancer: a matched-case control study. Laryngoscope 2004, 114:2182–2186.

[25] Malchoff CD, Sarfarazi M, Tendler B, Forouhar F, Whalen G, Joshi V, Arnold A, Malchoff DM. Papillary thyroid carcinoma associated with papillary renal neoplasia: genetic linkage analysis of a distinct heritable tumor syndrome. JCEM 2000, 85:1758-1764.

[26] Suh I, Filetti S, Vriens MR, Guerrero MA, Tumino S, Wong M, Shen WT, Kebebew E, Duh QY, Clark OH. Distinct loci on chromosome 1q21 and 6q22 predispose to familial nonmedullary thyroid cancer: a SNP array-based linkage analysis of 38 families. Surgery 2009, 146:1073-80.

[27] He H, Nagy R, Liyanarachchi S, Jiao H, Li W, Suster S, Kere J, de la Chapelle A. A susceptibility locus for papillary thyroid carcinoma on chromosome 8q24. Cancer Res. 2009, 69:625-31.

[28] Cavaco BM, Batista PF, Sobrinho LG, Leite V. Mapping a new familial thyroid epithelial neoplasia susceptibility locus to chromosome 8p23.1-p22 by high-density single-nucleotide polymorphism genome-wide linkage analysis. JCEM 2008, 93:4426-30.

[29]   Bignell GR, Canzian F, Shayeghi M, Stark M, Shugart YY, Biggs P, Mangion J, Hamoudi R, Rosenblatt J, Buu P, Sun S, Stoffer SS, Goldgar DE, Romeo G, Houlston RS, Narod SA, Stratton MR, Foulkes WD. Familial nontoxic multinodular thyroid goiter locus maps to chromosome 14q but does not account for familial nonmedullary thyroid cancer. American Journal of Human Genetics 1997, 61:1123–1130.

[30]   Neumann S, Willgerodt H, Ackermann F, Reske A, Jung M, Reis A, Paschke R. Linkage of familial euthyroid goiter to the multinodular goiter-1 locus and exclusion of the candidate genes thyroglobulin, thyroperoxidase, and Na+/I- symporter. JCEM 1999, 84:3750-56.

[31]   Lesueur F, Stark M, Tocco T. Genetic heterogeneity in familial nonmedullary thyroid carcinoma: exclusion of linkage to RET, MNG1, and TCO in 56 families. JCEM 1999, 84:2157–2162.

[32]   McKay JD, Thompson D, Lesueur F, Stankov K, Pastore A, Watfah C, Strolz S, Riccabona G, Moncayo R, Romeo G, Goldgar DE. Evidence for interaction between the TCO and NMTC1 loci in familial non-medullary thyroid cancer. J Med Genet. 2004, 41:407-12.

[33]   Capezzone M, Cantara S, Marchisotta S, Filetti S, Ronga G, Durante C, De Santi MM, Rossi B, Pacini F. Short telomeres, telomerase reverse transcriptase gene amplification, and increased telomerase activity in the blood of familial papillary thyroid cancer patients. JCEM 2008, 93:3950-7.

[34]   Capezzone M, Cantara S, Marchisotta S, Busonero G, Formichi C, Benigni M, Capuano S, Toti P, Pazaitou-Panayiotou K, Caruso G, Carli AF, Palummo N, Pacini F. Telomere length in neoplastic and nonneoplastic tissues of patients with familial and sporadic papillary thyroid cancer. JCEM 2011, 96:E1852-6.

[35]   Gisselsson D Mitotic instability in cancer: is there method in the madness? Cell Cycle. 2005, 4:1007-10.

[36]   Cantara S, Pisu M, Frau DV, Caria P, Dettori T, Capezzone M, Captano S, Vanni R, Pacini F. Telomere abnormalities and chromosome fragility in patients affected by familial papillary thyroid cancer. JCEM April, 2012 [Epub ahead of print].

[37]   Jendrzejewski J, Tomsic J, Lozanski G, Labanowska J, He H, Liyanarachchi S, Nagy R, Ringel MD, Kloos RT, Heerema NA, de la Chapelle A. Telomere length and telomerase reverse transcriptase gene copy number in patients with papillary thyroid carcinoma. JCEM 2011, 96:E1876-80.

[38]   Ngan ES, Lang BH, Liu T, Shum CK, So MT, Lau DK, Leon TY, Cherny SS, Tsai SY, Lo CY, Khoo US, Tam PK, Garcia-Barceló MM. A germline mutation (A339V) in thyroid transcription factor-1 (TITF-1/NKX2.1) in patients with multinodular goiter and papillary thyroid carcinoma. J Natl Cancer Inst. 2009, 101:162-75.

[39]   Cantara S, Capuano S, Formichi C, Pisu M, Capezzone M, Pacini F. Lack of germline A339V mutation in thyroid transcription factor-1 (TITF-1/NKX2.1) gene in familial papillary thyroid cancer. Thyroid Res. 2010, 3:4.

*Send Orders for Reprints on reprints@benthamscience.net*

# CHAPTER 6

# Thyroid Cancer of Parafollicular Origin: Medullary Carcinoma

## Maria G. Castagna[*]

*Section of Endocrinology & Metabolism, Department of Medical, Surgical and Neurological Sciences University of Siena, Siena, Italy*

**Abstract:** Medullary thyroid carcinoma is a tumor of the parafollicular C cells which accounts approximately 3% of thyroid cancer. It may occur as sporadic form or hereditary cancer both alone or associated with syndromes. In this chapter, epidemiology, genetic, diagnosis and treatment of medullary thyroid cancer will be discussed.

**Keywords:** Medullary thyroid cancer, MEN2A, MEN2B, RET point mutations.

## INTRODUCTION

Medullary thyroid carcinoma (MTC) is a rare tumor of the thyroid parafollicular C cells accounting for approximately 3% of thyroid cancer [1].

Macroscopically, MTC presents as a firm nodule indistinguishable from other thyroid carcinomas [2, 3]. At histological examination, classic MTC consists of areas of spindle-shaped, round or polygonal cells separated by stroma. The nuclei are uniform in shape with rare mitotic figures. Cytoplasm is eosinophilic with a finely granular manifestation. Amyloid deposits are seen in 60 to 80 % of tumors and calcitonin is positive at immunochemistry (100% of the cases). Familial

---

[*]**Address correspondence to Maria G. Castagna:** Section of Endocrinology & Metabolism, Department of Internal Medicine, Endocrinology & Metabolism and Biochemistry, University of Siena, Siena, Italy; E-mail: m.g.castagna@ao-siena.toscana.it

MTCs are usually bilateral and multicentric, while sporadic MTC usually presents as single tumor. Clinical neck lymph-node metastases, are detected in at least 50% of patients [4, 5].

In MTC, neoplastic C cells retain the characteristic to release calcitonin (CT), a calcium lowering hormone which increases over 10 pg/ml [6, 7]. In some patients, basal CT may be normal but will rise after pentagastrin stimulation [6].

## GENETICS OF MEDULLARY THYROID CARCINOMA

Hereditary MTC originates from germline autosomal dominat mutations in RET proto-oncogene [8-12]. Mutations causing MEN 2A affect, in the majority of cases, the extracellular domain of the protein at codons 609, 611, 618, 620 (exon 10) and, at codon 634 (exon 11). In approximately 95 % of patients with MEN 2B a single mutation at codon 918 of exon 16 has been found [12]. In about half of FMTC kindred, codons 10, 13 and 14 are affected. Only in a limited number of families, mutations affect codons in exon 11 and 15 [12].

Recently, a high prevalence of RAS mutations was reported in RET-negative sporadic MTC, suggesting an alternative genetic event in MTC tumorigenesis. In these studies, RET negative samples were identified to be positive for mutations of H-and K-RAS whereas no mutations in NRAS or BRAF were found [13, 14]. RAS mutations in MTC have been demonstrated to be mutually exclusive with RET mutations by exome sequencing analysis [15-16].

## CLINICAL SYNDROMES

MTC is mostly sporadic, but a hereditary form is found in 20-30 % of the cases [17]. This form, the Multiple Endocrine Neoplasia (MEN) syndrome type 2, is characterized by MTC together with pheochromocytoma and hyperparathyroidism (MEN 2A) or MTC in combination with pheochromocytoma, multiple mucosal neuromas, and marfanoid habitus (MEN 2B). The occurrence of familial MTC (FMTC), in the absence of other cancer is also possible (Table **1**).

**Table 1:** Clinical presentation of familial medullary thyroid carcinoma

|  | FMTC | MEN 2A | MEN 2B |
|---|---|---|---|
| MTC | 100% | 100% | 100% |
| C-cell hyperpasia | 100% | 100% | 100% |
| Pheochromocytoma | 0% | 50% | 50% |
| Hyperparathyroidism | 0% | 30% | 0% |
| Lichen Amyloidosis | 0% | <10% | 0% |
| Marfanoid habitus | 0% | 0% | ~100% |
| Intestinal ganglioneuromatosis | 0% | 0% | ~90% |
| Mucosal neuromas | 0% | 0% | ~80% |

## SPORADIC MEDULLARY THYROID CARCINOMA

Sporadic cancer accounts up to 80% of all cases of medullary thyroid cancer and can be diagnosed with the help of FNAC. Nevertheless, cytology may be confusing and, in these cases, positive immunocytochemical staining for CT and/or CT measurement in the washout fluid of FNA will confirm the diagnosis [18, 19]. Increased serum levels of CT are almost diagnostic of MTC (>10 pg/mL). For this reason, routine measurement of serum CT in nodular thyroid disorders has been advocated by authoritative European centres for the detection of MTC [20, 21].

## MULTIPLE ENDOCRINE NEOPLASIA TYPE 2A

MEN 2A is a syndrome associated with MTC (100% of patients), pheochromo-cytoma (60% of patients) and hyperparathyroidism (20-30%). A pruritic and hyper pigmented skin lesion on the upper portion of the back has been found in several kindreds. Hirschsprung's disease has been observed in a few families with MEN 2A.

## MULTIPLE ENDOCRINE NEOPLASIA TYPE 2B

MEN2B is a syndrome associated with MTC, pheochromocytoma, ganglioneuromatosis, marfanoid features and skeletal abnormalities [22]. MTC occurring within MEN 2B is the most aggressive form and occurs usually before 5-10 years of age. Mucosal neuromas occur on the distal portion of the tongue, on the lips, throughout the intestinal tract and sometimes in the urinary tract. Hypertrophy of corneal nerves is frequent. Marfanoid features include long, thin extremities, an altered upper-to-lower body ratio and ligament hyperlaxity. Skeletal abnormalities include slipped femoral epiphysis and pectus excavatum.

## INITIAL TREATMENT FOR PATIENTS WITH MEDULLARY THYROID CARCINOMA

The preoperative laboratory exams should include basal serum CT, CEA, calcium and plasma metanephrines and normetanephrines, or 24-hour urine collection for metanephrines and normetanephrines. Preoperative instrumental imaging include neck US in all patients whereas preoperative chest CT, neck CT and three-phase contrast enhanced multidetector liver CT or contrast-enhanced MRI should be performed in patients with documented lymph node metastases or with serum CT >400 pg/ml [17].

## PROPHYLACTIC THYROIDECTOMY IN MEN 2 GENE CARRIERS

Given the high chance of developing MTC at some point during life, children carring RET gene mutations should undergo prophylactic thyroidectomy before age 5 (MEN 2A/FMTC) or within the first year of life (MEN 2B) [17].

In RET mutation-positive patients, screening for phemocromocytoma include annual plasma metanephrines and normetanephrines, or 24-hour urine collection for metanephrines and normetanephrines beginning by age 8 years in carriers of RET mutation associated with MEN 2B and codons 630 and 634, and by age 20 years in carriers of other MEN 2A RET mutations. Patients with RET mutation associated only with FMTC should be screened periodically from the age of 20 years. Screening for hyperparathyroidism should be performed.

## POST OPERATIVE MANAGEMENT

After total thyroidectomy, thyroxine is given to achieve normal serum TSH levels. Measurements of serum CT, 2-3 months post-operatively, is important to detect persistent or recurrent disease [17, 23] (Table **2**). Undetectable basal and stimulated serum CT levels indicate a complete remission [24]. Serum CT should be measured every 6 months for the first 2-3 years and annually thereafter [25].

On the contrary, if basal serum CT is detectable or becomes detectable after stimulation, the disease is persistent.

**Table 2:** Follow-up of MTC patients after surgery, according to the results of serum CT measurement [14]

| CT levels after initial surgery (2-3 months after) | | |
|---|---|---|
| Undetectable CT | Detectable CT (≤150 pg/ml) | Detectable CT (>150 pg/ml) |
| CT measurement every 6 months for 2-3 years and annually thereafter | Neck US±FNAB: **If positive**: therapy **If negative**: serum CT every 6 months (to evaluate DT) ± imaging | Neck US± additional imaging: **If positive**: therapy **If negative**: serum CT every 6 months (to evaluate DT) and imaging |

## TREATMENT OF LOCAL AND REGIONAL RECURRENCES

Whenever feasible, surgery is the treatment of choice for local and regional recurrences. The extent of surgery will be dictated by precise localization of the recurrence determined by complete pre-operative work-up, type of initial surgical procedures performed, and the nature of the relapse. In the absence of known distant metastases, EBRT of the neck and mediastinum may be indicated after reintervention, particularly when serum CT remains elevated.

## TREATMENT OF METASTATIC DISEASE

Distant metastases are the main reason of death in MTC subjects. In half of the cases, they are present from the beginning and often simultaneously affect different organs (*i.e.,* liver, lungs and bones). Management is oriented toward eradication or stabilization of the lesions [26]. Systemic chemotherapy with dacarbazine, fluorouracil and doxorubicin (alone or in combination) have shown only partial responses [27-35].

## CONFLICT OF INTEREST

The author confirms that she has no conflicts of interest.

## ACKNOWLEDGEMENTS

Declared none.

## DISCLOSURE

Part of this chapter has been previously published in Clinical Oncology Volume 22, Issue 6, August 2010, Pages 475–485.

## REFERENCES

[1]     Aschebrook-Kilfoy B, Ward MH, Sabra MM, Devesa SS. Thyroid cancer incidence patterns in the United States by histologic type, 1992-2006. Thyroid. 2011, 21:125-34.

[2]     Hedinger C., Williams E.D., Sobin L.H. Histological typing of thyroid tumours. 2ndEd n11 of International classification of tumours. Berlin, Germany: Springer-Verlag, 1988.

[3]     LiVolsi VA. C cell hyperplasia/neoplasia. J Clin Endocrinol Metab. 1997, 82:39-41.

[4]     Moley JF, DeBenedetti MK. Patterns of nodal metastases in palpable medullary thyroid carcinoma: recommendations for extent of node dissection. Ann Surg. 1999, 229:880-7.

[5]     Scollo C, Baudin E, Travagli JP, Caillou B, Bellon N, Leboulleux S, Schlumberger M. Rationale for central and bilateral lymph node dissection in sporadic and hereditary medullary thyroid cancer. J Clin Endocrinol Metab. 2003, 88:2070-5.

[6]     Baloch Z, Carayon P, Conte-Devolx B, Demers LM, Feldt-Rasmussen U, Henry JF, LiVosli VA, Niccoli-Sire P, John R, Ruf J, Smyth PP, Spencer CA, Stockigt JR; Guidelines Committee, National Academy of Clinical Biochemistry. Laboratory medicine practice guidelines. Calcitonin and RET proto-oncogene mesaurements. Thyroid 2003, 13:68-79.

[7]     Motté P, Vauzelle P, Gardet P, Ghillani P, Caillou B, Parmentier C, Bohuon C, Bellet D. Construction and clinical validation of a sensitive and specific assay for serum mature calcitonin using monoclonal anti-peptide antibodies. Clin Chim Acta 1988, 174:35-54.

[8]     Lois M. Mulligan, John B. J. Kwok, Catherine S. Healey, Mark J. Elsdon, Charis Eng, Emily Gardner, Donald R. Love, Sara E. Mole, Julie K. Moore, Laura Papi, Margaret A. Ponder, Hakan Telenius, Alan Tunnacliffe & Bruce A. J. Ponder. Germ-line mutations of the RET proto-oncogene in multiple endocrine neoplasia type 2A. Nature 1993, 363:458-60.

[9]     Robert M. W. Hofstra, Rudy M. Landsvater, Isabella Ceccherini, Rein P. Stulp, Tineke Stelwagen, Yin Luo, Barbara Pasini, Jo W. M. Hoppener, Hans Kristian Ploos van Amstel, Giovanni Romeo, Cornells J. M. Lips & Charles H. C. M. Buys. A mutation in the RET proto-oncogene associated with multiple endocrine neoplasia type 2B and sporadic medullary thyroid carcinoma. Nature 1994, 367:375-6.

[10]    Lois M. Mulligan, Charis Eng, Catherine S. Healey, David Clayton, John B.J. Kwok, Emily Gardner, Margaret A. Ponder, Andrea Frilling, Charles E. Jackson, Hendrik Lehnert, Hartmut P.H. Neumann, Stephen N. Thibodeau & Bruce A.J. Ponder. Specific mutations of the RET proto-oncogene are related to disease phenotype in MEN 2A and FMTC. Nat Genet 1994, 6:70-4.

[11]    Santoro M, Carlomagno F, Romano A, Bottaro DP, Dathan NA, Grieco M. *et al.* Activation of RET as a dominant transforming gene by germline mutations of MEN2A and MEN2B. Science 1995, 267:381-3.

[12]    Eng C, Clayton D, Schuffenecker I, Lenoir G, Cote G, Gagel RF, Ploos van Amstel HK, Lips CJM, Nishisho I, Takai SI, Marsh DJ, Robinson BG, Frank-Raue K, Raue F, Xue F, Noll WW, Romei C, Pacini F, Fink M, Niederle B, Zedenius J, Nordenskjöld M, Komminoth P, Hendy GN, Gharib H, Thibodeau SN, Lacroix A, Frilling A, Ponder BAJ, Mulligan LM,. The relationship between specific RET proto-oncogene mutations and

disease phenotype in multiple endocrine neoplasia type 2. International RET mutation consortium analysis. JAMA 1996, 276:1575-9.

[13]   Moura MM, Cavaco BM, Pinto AE, Leite V. High prevalence of RAS mutations in RET-negative sporadic medullary thyroid carcinomas. Clin Endocrinol Metab. 2011, 96:E863-8.

[14]   Boichard A, Croux L, Al Ghuzlan A, Broutin S, Dupuy C, Leboulleux S, Schlumberger M, Bidart JM, Lacroix L. Somatic RAS mutations occur in a large proportion of sporadic RET-negative medullary thyroid carcinomas and extend to a previously unidentified exon. JCEM 2012, 97:E2031-5.

[15]   Ciampi R, Mian C, Fugazzola L, Cosci B, Romei C, Barollo S, Cirello V, Bottici V, Marconcini G, Rosa PM, Borrello MG, Basolo F, Ugolini C, Materazzi G, Pinchera A, Elisei R. Evidence of a low prevalence of RAS mutations in a large medullary thyroid cancer series. Thyroid. 2013, 23:50-7.

[16]   Agrawal N, Jiao Y, Sausen M, Leary R, Bettegowda C, Roberts NJ, Bhan S, Ho AS, Khan Z, Bishop J, Westra WH, Wood LD, Hruban RH, Tufano RP, Robinson B, Dralle H, Toledo SP, Toledo RA, Morris LG, Ghossein RA, Fagin JA, Chan TA, Velculescu VE, Vogelstein B, Kinzler KW, Papadopoulos N, Nelkin BD, Ball DW. Exomic sequencing of medullary thyroid cancer reveals dominant and mutually exclusive oncogenic mutations in RET and RAS. JCEM 2013, 98:E364-9.

[17]   American Thyroid Association (ATA) Guidelines Taskforce on Thyroid Nodules and Differentiated Thyroid Cancer, Cooper DS, Doherty GM, Haugen BR, Kloos RT, Lee SL, Mandel SJ, Mazzaferri EL, McIver B, Pacini F, Schlumberger M, Sherman SI, Steward DL, Tuttle RM. Medullary thyroid cancer: management guidelines of the American Thyroid Association. Thyroid 2009, 19:565-612.

[18]   Schlumberger M and Pacini F. Thyroid tumors. Chapter 18, pp. 313-340. Edition Nucleon, Paris, 2006.

[19]   Boi F, Maurelli I, Pinna G, Atzeni F, Piga M, Lai ML, Mariotti S. Calcitonin measurement in wash-out fluid from fine needle aspiration of neck masses in patients with primary and metastatic medullary thyroid carcinoma. J Clin Endocrinol Metab 2007, 92:2115-8.

[20]   Kudo T, Miyauchi A, Ito Y, Takamura Y, Amino N, Hirokawa M. Diagnosis of medullary thyroid carcinoma by calcitonin measurement in fine-needle aspiration biopsy specimens. Thyroid 2007, 17:635-8.

[21]   Pacini F, Fontanelli M, Fugazzola L, Elisei R, Romei C, Di Coscio G, Miccoli P, Pinchera A. Routine measurement of serum calcitonin in nodular thyroid diseases allows the preoperative diagnosis of unsuspected sporadic medullary thyroid carcinoma. J Clin Endocrinol Metab 1994, 78:826-9.

[22]   Elisei R, Bottici V, Luchetti F, Di Coscio G, Romei C, Grasso L, Miccoli P, Iacconi P, Basolo F, Pinchera A, Pacini F. Impact of routine measurement of serum calcitonin on the diagnosis and outcome of medullary thyroid cancer: experience in 10,864 patients with nodular thyroid disorders. J Clin Endocrinol Metab 2004, 89:163-8.

[23]    Gagel RF, Jackson CE, Block MA, Feldman ZT, Reichlin S, Hamilton BP, Tashjian AH Jr. Age-related probability of development of hereditary medullary thyroid carcinoma. J Pediatr 1982, 101:941-6.

[24]    Brandi ML, Gagel RF, Angeli A, Bilezikian JP, Beck-Peccoz P, Bordi C *et al.*, Guidelines for diagnosis and therapy of MEN type 1 and type 2. J Clin Endocrinol Metab 2001, 86:5658-71.

[25]    Stepanas AV, Samaan NA, Hill CS Jr, Hickey RC. Medullary thyroid carcinoma: importance of serial serum calcitonin measurement. Cancer 1979, 43:825-37.

[26]    Machens A, Schneyer U, Holzhausen HJ, Dralle H. Prospects of remission in medullary thyroid carcinoma according to basal calcitonin level. J Clin Endocrinol Metab 2005, 90:2029-34.

[27]    Franc S, Niccoli-Sire P, Cohen R, Bardet S, Maes B, Murat A, Krivitzky A, Modigliani E; French Medullary Study Group (GETC). Complete surgical lymph node resection does not prevent authentic recurrences of medullary thyroid carcinoma. Clin Endocrinol 2001, 55:403-9.

[28]    Laure Giraudet A, Al Ghulzan A, Aupérin A, Leboulleux S, Chehboun A, Troalen F, Dromain C, Lumbroso J, Baudin E, Schlumberger M. Progression of medullary thyroid carcinoma: assessment with calcitonin and carcinoembryonic antigen doubling times. Eur J Endocrinol. 2008, 158:239-46.

[29]    Scherübl H, Raue F, Ziegler R.Combination chemotherapy of advanced medullary and differentiated thyroid cancer. Phase II study. J Cancer Res Clin Oncol 1990, 116:21-3.

[30]    Orlandi F, Caraci P, Berruti A, Puligheddu B, Pivano G, Dogliotti L, Angeli A. Chemotherapy with dacarbazine and 5-fluorouracil in advanced medullary thyroid cancer. Ann Oncol 1994, 5:763-5.

[31]    Wu LT, Averbuch SD, Ball DW, de Bustros A, Baylin SB, McGuire WP 3rd.Treatment of advanced medullary thyroid carcinoma with a combination of cyclophosphamide, vincristine, and dacarbazine. Cancer 1994, 73:432-6.

[32]    Schlumberger M, Abdelmoumene N, Delisle MJ, Couette JE Treatment of advanced medullary thyroid cancer with an alternating combination of 5 FU-streptozocin and 5 FU-dacarbazine. The Groupe d'Etude des Tumeurs a Calcitonine (GETC). Br J Cancer 1995, 71:363-5.

[33]    Di Bartolomeo M, Bajetta E, Bochicchio AM, Carnaghi C, Somma L, Mazzaferro V, Visini M, Gebbia V, Tumolo S, Ballatore P. A phase II trial of dacarbazine, fluorouracil and epirubicin in patients with neuroendocrine tumours. A study by the Italian Trials in Medical Oncology (I.T.M.O.) Group. Ann Oncol 1995, 6:77-9.

[34]    Petursson SR. Metastatic medullary thyroid carcinoma. Complete response to combination chemotherapy with dacarbazine and 5-fluorouracil. Cancer 1988, 62:1899-903.

[35]    Bajetta E, Rimassa L, Carnaghi C, Seregni E, Ferrari L, Di Bartolomeo M, Regalia E, Cassata A, Procopio G, Mariani L. 5-Fluorouracil, dacarbazine, and epirubicin in the treatment of patients with neuroendocrine tumors. Cancer 1998, 83:372-8.

# CHAPTER 7

# Tyrosine Kinase Inhibitor and Target Therapy

**Brilli Lucia**[*]

*Section of Endocrinology & Metabolism, Department of Medical, Surgical and Neurological Sciences University of Siena, Siena, Italy*

**Abstract:** "Tyrosine kinase inhibitors" (TKI) are small molecules responsible for selectively inhibiting cellular pathways involved in cell proliferation or migration. These molecules have been developed as alternative therapy for refractory or minimal responsive cancers to standard treatments. In this chapter, TKI currently used for anaplastic thyroid cancer, medullary thyroid cancer and/or refractory differentiated thyroid cancer will be described.

**Keywords:** Tyrosine kinase, Tyrosine Kinase Inhibitors (TKI), growth factor receptors.

## INTRODUCTION

An important challenge in thyroid cancer treatment is represented by patients with tumours unresponsive to conventional treatments. Differentiated thyroid cancer (DTC), in most cases, is efficiently cured by standard treatment (total thyroidectomy, radioiodine ablation (RAI) and l-thyroxine suppressive therapy). However, around 10-15% of DTCs become refractory to radioactive iodine during the course of disease, leading to a decrease in survival. In the case of medullary thyroid cancer (MTC), the only effective therapeutic procedure is surgery and, for metastatic MTC, the general survival rate is 25% at 5 years. Finally, all cases of

---

[*]**Address correspondence to Brilli Lucia:** Section of Endocrinology & Metabolism, Department of Internal Medicine, Endocrinology & Metabolism and Biochemistry, University of Siena, Siena, Italy;
E-mail: luciabrilli@alice.it

anaplastic thyroid cancers have an extremely poor prognosis with a survival rate that rarely exceed 6-12 months and no effective treatment is available. In addition, for these cancers, external beam radiotherapy or chemotherapy are minimally effective. For all these situations, new treatment modalities are required.

In the last decade, significant progress has been made in the understanding mutations responsible for thyroid multi-step cancerogenesis. These alterations involve mainly kinase oncoproteins or protein ubiquitary-?? --expressed involved in controlling cell proliferation and migration [1] (see chapter 3 of this eBook).

In the last decade, new compounds have been produced that target these activated oncoproteins. The majority of these drugs inhibit tyrosine kinases, so in general we refer to this new class of drugs as "Tyrosine kinase inhibitors" (TKI). TKI are small molecules able to pass through cell membranes due to their hydrophobic properties (in contrast to monoclonal antibodies that interact only towards targets on the cell surface or secreted proteins). Most of the TKI are directed towards the ATP-binding site of the kinases, thereby inhibiting phosphorylation of the kinase and downstream substrates. The first tyrosine kinase inhibitor (TKI) approved for cancer treatment was imatinib, used to treat Philadelphia chromosome/BCR-ABL (+) chronic myelogenous leukaemia [2]. Since then, many other compounds have reached clinical approval or are still under investigation in clinical trials for haematological and solid tumours.

Unfortunately cancer cells, due to their genetic instability, develop new mutations that allow an escape from the TKI therapy. Inhibition of multiple genes or pathways is required to reach a clinical response, and for this reason, trials are ongoing to evaluate different drugs targeting different TKs in combination.

## CHALLENGES

Targeted therapy is usually better tolerated than chemotherapy but it has to be used chronically. The severity of adverse events is established, by convention, according to the Common Terminology Criteria for Adverse Events (CTCAE) reported by the National Cancer Institute. Side effects are rarely so severe that therapy is discontinued. More commonly, it may be necessary to reduce the drug's dose and, only in few cases, it may be necessary to withdraw therapy for a short period until the side effects improve. The most common side effects are constitutional symptoms such as fatigue, asthenia and weight loss. Diarrhoea has also been frequently observed. Hypertension is frequently observed especially with VEGF inhibitors. Dermatological side effects often occur, including rash, xerosis, hand-foot skin reaction (HFSR), mucositis and alopecia. Normally, these events happen by 6 weeks of therapy and frequently in the first 2 weeks. No consensus exists concerning the treatment of these cases [3]. Another common side effect is an increase of serum TSH probably due to interference in thyroid hormone metabolism or a decrease in l-tyroxine absorption [4].

Resistance to TKI is a growing problem and it constitutes an important limitation to their use. Patient may be genetically resistant to treatment or may develop resistance during therapy. This phenomenon may be due to several mechanisms such as mutations that modify receptor-inhibitor interactions, amplification and/or overexpression of the TKI's targets or enhancement of pre-existing expression of alternative pro-angiogenic pathways that evade the activity of the drug [5].

Interestingly, resistance to one TKI does not imply a resistance to another one, so changing to another TKI after demonstration of resistance is advisable.

## TKI IN THYROID CANCER PATIENTS

Of the many compounds tested for thyroid cancer since 2005, only one compound has received approval by the FDA and EMA for the treatment of MTC patients, based on results recently published from a phase III trial in patients with advanced MTC [6].

The efficacy of TKI is assessed by imaging techniques such CT or MR according to Response Evaluation Criteria in Solid Tumours (RECIST) guidelines. Following these criteria, measurable lesions were identified as targets, up to 5 per organ and 10 in total, and the sum of their longest diameter (SLT) was recorded in each evaluation and compared to determine the objective drug response. Briefly, according to these criteria, a complete response (CR) is defined as a disappearance of all target lesions, a partial response (PR) as a reduction of SLT of more than 30%, progressive disease (PD) as an appearance of one or more new lesions or a clear progression of non-target lesions or an increase at least 20% in the SLT, taking as reference the smallest SLT recorded since the treatment started. Stable disease (SD is a condition between PR and PD).

However, RECIST criteria have some limitations. The most important is probably that, in particular cases, objective response may be underestimated since a lesion may not reduce in size but may instead have a change in tumour density that indicates a drug's efficacy. Moreover, the target lesions may not respond to the drug, whereas other lesions (classified as non-target) may show significant shrinkage but are not considered when defining a partial response.

## CLINICAL TRIALS

The following describes results obtained with TKIs for thyroid cancer treatment among randomized phase II/III trials:

*Motesanib* (AMG706): The first TKI used in a large prospective trial among patients with thyroid cancer was motesanib diphosphate, a drug with the ability to inhibit several tyrosine kinases, mainly the VEGF receptors 1, 2 and 3. After a Phase I study on patients with advanced solid cancers, where 3/7 patients with thyroid cancer obtained a partial response [7], an open-label multicentric phase II trial was performed starting at 125 mg/daily in patients with DTC and MTC with progressive disease or a symptomatic disease (diarrhoea) for MTC, according to the RECIST criteria. Among 93 patients with DTC, partial responses were confirmed in 14% and stable disease in 67%, with an estimate median progression free survival (mPFS) of 40 weeks [8]. In 91 patients with MTC, 2% had PR and 81% SD with an estimate mPFS of 12 months [9]. In these patients, lower baseline VEGF levels correlated with longer PFS [10].

*Sorafenib* (BAY 43-9006): is a multikinase inhibitor which acts against VEGFr2 and 3, PDGFr, RAF and RET kinases. It was initially tested in two phase II trials, at the dose of 400 mg twice a day. In the first study published [11] among 22 patients with DTC, a PR was obtained in 31% and a SD in the remaining group. In the Kloos' study among 41 PTC patients, long-lasting (>6 months) stable disease was achieved in 56% while a partial response was observed in 15%. Based on these excellent results, a multicenter double-blind phase III trial, in advanced/metastatic radiodine refractory DTC patients was instituted and is now in progress [12].

Sorafenib has shown poor activity in bone metastases and no effect on the induction of $^{131}$I uptake [13]. The drug has also been tested in MTC patients in a phase II trial [14]: one patient achieved partial response (7%) while 14 had stable disease (93%).

*Sunitinib* (SU011248): exerts its activity against RET, VEGFr, PDGFr and other TKr. In a phase II trial, it was given to patients with refractory thyroid cancer (50 mg daily), four weeks on and two weeks off with a PR in 14% and a SD in 68% [15]. De Souza *et al.* [16] tested sunitinib at the same dosage in 25 patients with MTC. Among 23 evaluable patients, partial response was achieved in 8 (35%), whereas 13 (57%) had stable disease. In another phase II trial, sunitinib was given to 33 iodine refractory DTC and MTC, with one complete response (3%), 10 partial responses (28%) and 16 patients (46%) with stable disease. Interestingly, the authors observed a significant association between decreased 18FDG-PET uptake and favourable RECIST response [17]. Ravaud *et al.* [18] carried out a phase II trial in 15 MTC patients. Among these, 2 had a confirmed partial response and 3 an unconfirmed partial response (33, 3%) whereas stable disease for ≥12 weeks was achieved in 4 (26.7%).

*Vandetanib* (ZD6474): Vandetanib is an oral, small molecule with an inhibitory effect on VEGFr2, RET and EGFr. It was tested in two open label phase II trials in metastastic hereditary MTC. In the first [19] with a daily dose of 300 mg, a confirmed partial response was achieved in 20% while a prolonged stable disease occurred in 53% of the patients. In the second trial by Robinson *et al.* [20], with a dosage of 100 mg daily, a partial response was reported in 16% patients and a prolonged stable disease in 53%. A phase III, double-blind, placebo-controlled trial randomized 331 patients with advanced MTC. The results of the study showed that treatment with vandetanib (300 mg once daily) significantly extended progression-free survival, the primary endpoint of the study. The objective response rate (ORR), a secondary endpoint, was 45% *versus* 13% across the two groups [6]. Based on these results, US Food and Drug Administration and the European Medicines Agency have recently accepted vandetanib for the treatment of advanced MTC patients with the trade name of Caprelsa®. Vandetanib was also administered in a phase II trial in advanced DTC patients obtaining a PFS of 11 months, *versus* 5.8 months of the placebo group [21].

Axitinib (AG-013736): is a selective inhibitor of VEGFr and PDGF-βr. After a pilot phase I trial [22] in patients with advanced solid tumours, a multicenter, single arm, phase II trial [23] was conducted in 60 subjects with advanced or metastatic thyroid cancer starting at a dose of 5 mg twice a day. Stable disease was obtained in 38% of the patients; PR was observed in 18% of the patients with MTC and 31% of the patients with DTC.

*Cabozantinib* (XL184): is an oral inhibitor of several TK receptors. The primary targets are VEGFR2, RET, c-KIT and MET. In a phase I trial [24] 29% of MTC patients with measurable disease achieved a partial response and 41%

had a best response of prolonged ($\geq$ 6 months) stable disease. Preliminary results of a phase III trial, comparing XL184 and placebo in 330 patients with progressive, metastatic MTC, showed a statistically significant median PFS prolongation of 7.2 months with a 1 year PFS rate of 47.3% [25]. Cabozantinib seems to have an anti-tumour activity also in DTC: indeed it has been recently tested in RAI-refractory metastatic DTC obtaining a confirmed partial response [26].

*Lenvatinib* (E7080): is a potent inhibitor of multiple receptor tyrosine kinases including VEGFR, FGFR1-4, RET and KIT. Lenvatinib was recently tested in a phase II trial for patients with advanced radioiodine (RAI)-refractory DTC and MTC, with a starting dose of 24 mg once daily. Preliminary data indicated that among 54 MTC patients [27], a confirmed PR was observed in 21 patients. Among 58 DTCpatients, the drug demonstrated an objective Response Rate (ORR) in 34 (59%) based on an updated investigator assessment [28].

*Pazopanib* (GW786034): is a molecule targeting VEGFr, PDGFr, c-KIT and other kinases. It has been tested at the daily dose of 800 mg in patients with metastatic, radioiodine-refractory DTC with a radiographically confirmed disease progression within 6 months before enrolment. Among 37 evaluable patients no one had a complete response, but 18 (49%) had a confirmed partial response. Average survival at 1 year was 81%, PFS at 1 year was 47% and median duration of PFS was 11.7 months. Pazopanib concentrations were significant higher in the 18 patients who obtained confirmed RECIST partial responses than in those who did not [29].

*Selumetinib* (AZD6244): this drug is an inhibitor of MEK, enzyme involved in the RAS/RAF/MEK/ERK pathway. Recently it has been used in patients with iodine-131 refractory papillary thyroid carcinoma with 3% of patients showing a PR and 66% patients maintaining stable disease [30].

## CONCLUSIONS

Treatment with TKI has led to encouraging results among patients with advanced differentiated and medullary thyroid cancer. In DTC patients, TKI therapy has been positive: partial responses were observed in 3-53% of patients and a stable disease was seen in around one-half of patients. Also in MTC, patients partial responses were seen in 2-39% of patients while a long-term stable disease response was observed in 41-53% of the cases. An important milestone was reached with the results obtained with the use of vandetanib. The drug significantly improved progression free survival with a good objective disease response and these results led to marketing authorization of vandetanib, with the trade name Caprelsa®.

Issues that are still open on the use of such therapies include drug resistance and toxicities. Future studies should be directed to strategies to overcome acquired resistance or to restore drug sensitivity. Improving molecular characterization of tumors may optimize the selection of patients for therapy and allow the identification of serum biomarkers that could predict clinical outcomes of drug therapy.

Regarding drug toxicities, it remains unknown chronic administration over time will lead to more side effects. Management of adverse events during therapy should be restricted to qualified persons who are skilled and accustomed to the management of complications. It would be advisable to define evidence-based strategies to follow patients during therapy.

In conclusion, based on current data, we recommend targeted therapy, possibly within clinical trials, in patients with advanced thyroid cancer refractory to conventional treatment and with progressive disease. For progressive and metastatic, vandetanib should be used as primary approach and only in case of resistance or drug intolerance should another TKI should be considered.

## CONFLICT OF INTEREST

The author confirms that she has no conflicts of interest.

## ACKNOWLEDGEMENTS

Declared none.

## REFERENCES

[1] Fagin JA, Mitsiades N. Molecular pathology of thyroid cancer: diagnostic and clinical implications. Best Pract Res Clin Endocrinol Metab. 2008, 22:955-69.

[2] Druker BJ, Guilhot F, O'Brien SG *ET AL*. Five-year follow-up of patients receiving imatinib for chronic myeloid leukemia. N Engl J Med. 2006, 355:2408-17.

[3] Lacouture ME, Wu S, Robert C *et al.* Evolving strategies for the management of hand-foot skin reaction associated with the multitargeted kinase inhibitors sorafenib and sunitinib. Oncologist. 2008, 13:1001-11.

[4] Brown RL. Tyrosine kinase inhibitor-induced hypothyroidism: incidence, etiology, and management. Target Oncol. 2011, 6:217-26.

[5] Sierra JR, Cepero V, Giordano S. Molecular mechanisms of acquired resistance to tyrosine kinase targeted therapy. Molecular Cancer 2010, 75:1476-4598.

[6] Wells SA Jr, Robinson BG, Gagel RF, Dralle H, Fagin JA, Santoro M, Baudin E, Elisei R, Jarzab B, Vasselli JR, Read J, Langmuir P, Ryan AJ, Schlumberger MJ.Vandetanib in patients with locally advanced or metastatic medullary thyroid cancer: a randomized, double-blind phase III trial.J Clin Oncol. 2012, 30:134-41.

[7] Rosen LS, Kurzrock R, Mulay M *et al.* Safety, pharmacokinetics, and efficacy of AMG 706, an oral multikinase inhibitor, in patients with advanced solid tumors. J Clin Oncol. 2007, 25:2369-76.

[8] Brilli L, Pacini F. Targeted therapy in refractory thyroid cancer: current achievements and limitations. Future Oncology. 2011, 7:657-668.

[9] Schlumberger MJ, Elisei R, Bastholt L *et al.* Phase II study of safety and efficacy of motesanib in patients with progressive or symptomatic, advanced or metastatic medullary thyroid cancer. J Clin Oncol. 2009, 27:3794-801.

[10] Bass MB, Sherman SI, Schlumberger M *et al.* Biomarkers as Predictors of Response to Treatment with Motesanib in Patients with Progressive Advanced Thyroid Cancer. J Clin Endocrinol Metab. 2010, 95:5018-27.

[11] Gupta-Abramson V, Troxel AB, Nellore A *et al.* Phase II trial of sorafenib in advanced thyroid cancer. J Clin Oncol. 2008, 26:4714-9.

[12]   Brose MS, Nutting CM, Sherman SI, Shong YKS, Smit JWA, Reike G, Chung J, Kalmus J, Christian Kappeler, and Martin Schlumberger. Rationale and design of decision: a double-blind, randomized, placebo-controlled phase III trial evaluating the efficacy and safety of sorafenib in patients with locally advanced or metastatic radioactive iodine (RAI)-refractory, differentiated thyroid cancer. BMC 2011, 11;11:349.

[13]   Hoftijzer H, Heemstra KA, Morreau H *et al.* Beneficial effects of sorafenib on tumor progression, but not on radioiodine uptake, in patients with differentiated thyroid carcinoma. Eur J Endocrinol. 2009, 161:923-31.

[14]   Lam ET, Ringel MD, Kloos RT *et al.* Phase II clinical trial of sorafenib in metastatic medullary thyroid cancer. J Clin Oncol. 2010, 28:2323-30.

[15]   Cohen EE, Needles BM, Cullen KJ *et al.* Phase II study of sunitinib in refractory thyroid cancer. Presented at: 2008 ASCO Annual Meeting. Abstract 6025. Chicago, USA, 30 May-3 June 2008.

[16]   De Souza JA, Busaidy N, Zimrin A *et al.* Phase II trial of sunitinib in medullary thyroid cancer (MTC). Presented at: 2010 ASCO Annual Meeting. Abstract 5504. Chicago, USA, 4-8 June 2010.

[17]   Carr LL, Mankoff D, Goulart BH *et al.* Phase II Study of Sunitinib in FDG-PET Positive, Differentiated Thyroid Cancer and Metastatic Medullary Carcinoma of Thyroid with Functional Imaging Correlation. Clin Cancer Res. 2010, 16:5260-8.

[18]   Ravaud A, De La Fouchardiére C, Asselineau J *et al.* Efficacy of sunitinib in Advanced Medullary Thyroid Carcinoma: Intermediate Results of phase II THYSU. The Oncologist. 2010, 15:212-213.

[19]   Wells SA Jr, Gosnell JE, Gagel RF *et al.* Vandetanib for the treatment of patients with locally advanced or metastatic hereditary medullary thyroid cancer. J Clin Oncol. 2010, 28:767-72.

[20]   Robinson BG, Paz-Ares L, Krebs A, Vasselli J, Haddad R. Vandetanib (100 mg) in patients with locally advanced or metastatic hereditary medullary thyroid cancer. J Clin Endocrinol Metab. 2010, 95:2664-71.

[21]   Leboulleux S, Bastholt L, Krause TM *et al.* Vandetanib in locally advanced or metastatic differentiated thyroid cancer (papillary or follicular; DTC): a randomized, double-blind Phase II trial. Presented at: 14th International Thyroid Congress. Oral Communication 023. Paris, 11-16 September 2010.

[22]   Rugo HS, Herbst RS, Liu G *et al.* Phase I trial of the oral antiangiogenesis agent AG-013736 in patients with advanced solid tumors: pharmacokinetic and clinical results. J Clin Oncol. 2005, 23:5474-83.

[23]   Cohen EE, Rosen LS, Vokes EE *et al.* Axitinib is an active treatment for all histologic subtypes of advanced thyroid cancer: results from a phase II study. J Clin Oncol 2008, 26:4708-13.

[24]   Kurzrock R, Sherman SI, Ball DW *et al.* Activity of XL184 (Cabozantinib), an oral tyrosine kinase inhibitor, in patients with medullary thyroid cancer. J Clin Oncol 2011, 29:2660-6.

[25]   Schoffski P, Elisei R, Muller S, Brose MS *et al.* An international, double-blind, randomized, placebo-controlled phase III trial (EXAM) of cabozantinib (XL184) in medullary thyroid carcinoma (MTC) patients (pts) with documented RECIST progression at baseline. J Clin Oncol 30, 2012 (suppl; abstr 5508).

[26]   Cabanillas ME, Brose MS, Ramies DA *et al.* Antitumor Activity of Cabozantinib (XL184) in a cohort of patients with differentiated thyroid cancer (DTC). J Clin Oncol 30, 2012 (suppl; abstr:5547)

[27]   Schlumberger M, jarzab B, Cabanillas M *et al.* A phase II trial of the multi-targeted kinase inhibitor lenvatinib (E7080) in advanced medullary thyroid cancer. J Clin Oncol 30, 2012 (suppl; abstr 5591).

[28]   Sherman SI, Jarzab B, Cabanillas ME *et al.* A phase II trail of the multitargeted kinase inhibitor E7080 in advanced radioiodine (RAI)-refractory differentiated thyroid cancer (DTC). J Clin Oncol 29: 2011 (suppl; abstr 5503)

[29]   Bible KC, Suman VJ, Molina JR *et al.* Efficacy of pazopanib in progressive, radioiodine-refractory, metastatic differentiated thyroid cancers: results of a phase 2 consortium study. Lancet Oncol. 2010, 11:962-972.

[30]   Hayes DN, Lucas AS, Tanvetyanon T, Krzyzanowska MK, Chung CH, Murphy BA, Gilbert J, Mehra R, Moore DT, Sheikh A, Hoskins J, Hayward MC, Zhao N, O'Connor W, Weck KE, Cohen RB, Cohen EE. Phase II efficacy and pharmacogenomic study of Selumetinib (AZD6244; ARRY-142886) in iodine-131 refractory papillary thyroid carcinoma with or without follicular elements. Clin Cancer Res. 2012, 18:2056-65.

# CHAPTER 8

## Potential Markers for the Diagnosis of Thyroid Cancer

### Silvia Cantara[*]

*Section of Endocrinology & Metabolism, Department of Internal Medicine, Endocrinology & Metabolism and Biochemistry, University of Siena, Siena, Italy*

**Abstract:** Some of the genetic alterations described in thyroid cancer, such as RET/PTC rearrangements, RAS point mutations and PAX8/PPARγ rearrangements, have also been found in benign lesions. The only exception is the point mutation V600E of BRAF oncogene, which is specific for the malignant histology. For this reason, researchers are seeking new markers expressed only by cancer tissues. Among these, telomerase activity and expression, together with miRNAs expression, have been proposed to be able to distinguish benign from malignant lesions both in tissues and FNAC samples with high specificity.

**Keywords:** miRNA, molecular diagnosis, telomerase, telomere.

## INTRODUCTION

Papillary thyroid carcinoma (PTC) and follicular thyroid carcinoma (FTC) are the most common types of thyroid cancers with a frequency of 80% and 11%, respectively [1]. Genomic alterations responsible for thyroid carcinomas are specific for different histological subtypes (see chapter 3). The most common of these mutations is an alteration in the BRAF oncogene, which is present in approximately 44% (29-83%) of PTCs [2, 3]. On the contrary, follicular adenomas and carcinomas contain PAX8-PPARgamma rearrangements [4, 5]. Activating mutations in RAS occur both in follicular adenomas and carcinomas,

---

[*]**Address correspondence to Silvia Cantara:** Section of Endocrinology & Metabolism, Department of Internal Medicine, Endocrinology & Metabolism and Biochemistry, University of Siena, Siena, Italy; E-mail: cantara@unisi.it

as well as in the follicular variant of PTC [6-8]. RET/PTC gene rearrangements occur in radiation-associated sporadic PTC as well as in follicular adenomas [9-11]. Although all these genetic changes contribute to the diagnosis of malignant thyroid lesions, with the exception of BRAF point mutation, they have also been found in benign lesions. There is a need to find other marker specific for thyroid malignancy. Here we review some of the candidates.

## TELOMERASE ACTIVITY AND EXPRESSION

Telomeres are non-coding regions at the end of chromosomes consisting of several copies of TTAGGG sequence that stabilize chromosomes during cell division. Telomeres are preserved by telomerase, a specialized ribonucleoprotein complex that includes an RNA template (TERC) and a reverse transcriptase catalytic subunit (TERT) (Fig. **1**) [12].

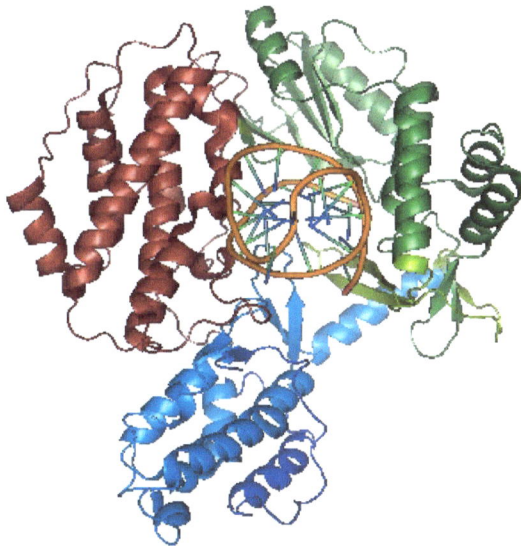

**Figure 1:** Hypothetical model of *Tetrahymena castaneum* TERT elaborated with PyMol program. The N-terminal domain is in blue and the telomerase RNA binding domain (TRBD) in light blue. The position of fingers is in light green and the position of palm is in dark green (together they form the core domain). Thumb, which corresponds to C-terminal domain, is in red. Telomere DNA is shown bound to the protein.

Telomeres are progressively lost with each cell division due to incomplete replication of the ends of linear DNA. When telomeres reach a critically short length, the cells undergo senescence and apoptosis. In the case of altered checkpoint mechanisms, genomic instability occurs and begins a period called "crisis", characterized by cycles of chromosome breakage and fusion that contribute to the acquisition of further genetic alterations [12]. During "crisis", most of the cells die by apoptosis, but a few cells can survive and stabilize short telomeres through telomerase activity that facilitates cell immortalization which is linked to tumour development [13] (Fig. **2**).

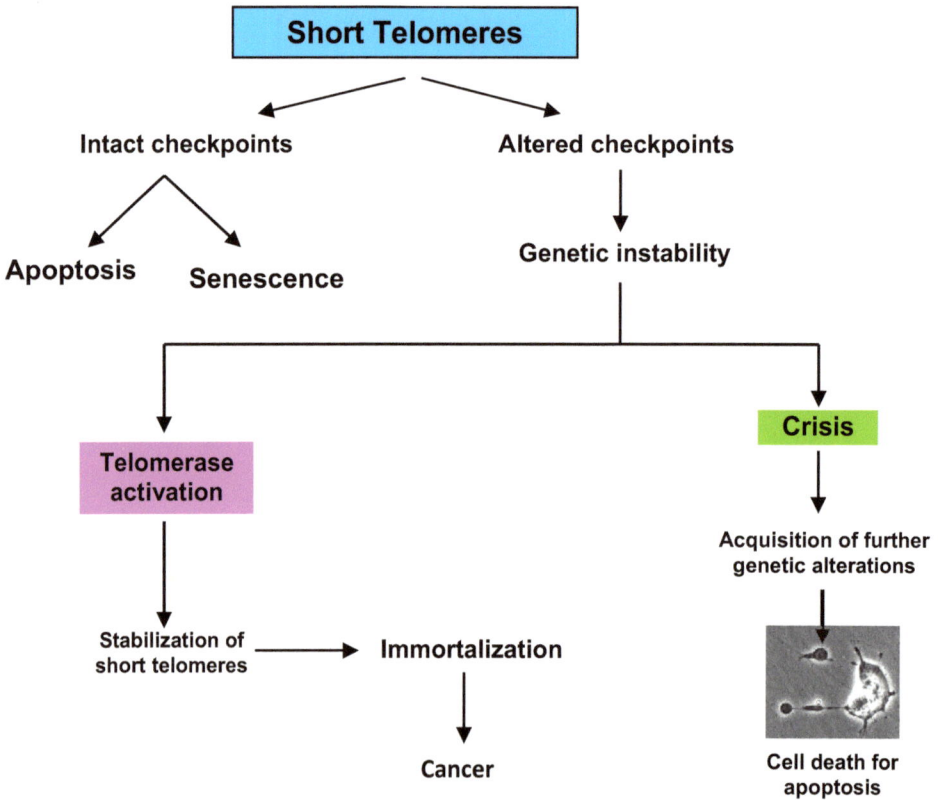

**Figure 2:** Schematic representation of the process leading to cell immortalization.

Studies on thyroid tissues: Telomerase expression and activity is low or absent in most human somatic tissues including thyroid cells. On the contrary, among thyroid cancer, increased telomerase activity or expression was found in all histological types,(papillary, follicular, medullary and anaplastic), with large variations in different series, but more than 50% of the samples [14-33]. Among these studies, Umbrich *et al.* [21] in 1997 first demonstrated the presence of telomerase activity (TA) in follicular thyroid carcinomas suggesting that TA may represent a potential diagnostic marker for this particular histological type of thyroid cancer. In a different paper, TA was found in papillary thyroid carcinomas (PTC), but not in benign adenomas, follicular carcinomas, or most normal thyroid tissues (14). Telomerase expression was also associated with thyroid carcinoma. Takano *et al.* [31] showed the presence of high levels of hTERT mRNA expression in anaplastic thyroid specimen and cell lines. Interestingly, a recent paper [32] reported that the down regulation of microRNA miR-138 expression may partially contribute to the gain of hTERT protein expression in anaplastic thyroid cancer. Some studies [17, 25, 26, 33] showed that telomerase expression correlated significantly with clinical stage. In addition, Foukakis *et al.* [34] evaluated 10 potential gene markers of malignancy in a panel of 75 follicular tumours of different clinical behaviour and identified two genes, *TERT* and *TTF3*, whose combination was able to distinguish adenomas and low grade follicular carcinomas from aggressive follicular carcinomas.

Experiences on FNAC: TA and telomerase expression have been evaluated also in FNAC as possible marker to increase FNAC diagnostic accuracy [35-41] with contrasting results. In two studies [35, 38] a clear difference in detectable TA between FNAC samples that were histologically confirmed as malignant and those that were diagnosed as benign lesions, is reported. On the contrary, other authors [36, 39] concluded that the detection of TA in cytological specimens does not add practical diagnostic information to distinguish between benign and malignant lesions. Guerra *et al.* [40] proposed that if a 10-Unit cut off as level of TA is established, detectable TA would be confined to thyroid carcinomas only, and could be a useful marker in the diagnosis of thyroid cancer, especially in indeterminate FNAC cases.

Several papers also reported that RT-PCR for hTERT gene may be useful as a preoperative method for the evaluation of thyroid lesions [24, 28, 30, 41].

**Methods for the Analysis of Telomerase Activity**

1) *ELISA kit.* An ELISA is a biochemical technique used to detect the presence of an antibody or an antigen in a sample. Several kits have been developed by different companies. Generally it is important to evaluate protein concentrations and standardize the amounts for each sample. Telomeric repeats are added to a biotin-labeled primer by telomerase, followed by the amplification of the elongation product by PCR. The PCR product is then denatured, bound to a Strept/Avidin coated 96-well plate, and hybridized to a DIG labeled telomeric repeat-specific probe. An antibody to DIG, conjugated to peroxidase, is subsequently bound to DIG and visualized by a colorimetric reaction. Sample absorbance is then measured at the appropriate wavelength using an ELISA plate reader [42]. Internal positive and negative controls are usually provided by the kits.

2) *Telomere Repeat Amplification Protocol (TRAP).* The TRAP assay was described by Kim *et al.* [43] in 1994. The principle of the assay is to measure enzymatic activity of telomerase in a two-step experiment. In the first passage, the telomerase elongates a forward primer that simulates the telomere end. In the second part, a reverse primer, complementary to the telomere repeat, is added and a polymerase chain reaction is carried out. PCR products are then electrophoresed on a polyacrylamide gel previously stained in order to visualize the 6 bp ladder. Since the first protocol, several modifications have occurred, especially with the introduction of internal standard [15] which is necessary because some tissue samples contain an inhibitor

of polymerase, which may result in false-negative values and to permit relative quantification of enzyme activity.

## Methods to Measure Telomerase Expression

1) *Real time PCR.* Here we describe the method and primers used in our laboratory [42]. RNA is extracted and 1 µg for each sample is retro-transcribed into complementary cDNA. After, 30 ng/µl are used for Q-RT PCR in a mix containing 12.5 µl SYBER GREEN PCR Master Mix, 900 nM of each primers (primer forward 3'-ACGGCGACATGGAGAACAA-5', primer reverse 3'-CACTGTCTTCCGCAAGTTCAC-5') for a final volume of 25 µl. RNA quantity standards need to be added in order to produce a standard curves for final quantification. The thermal cycling profile is: 95° for 10 min followed by 35 cycles of 95°C for 15 s and 60°C for 1 min. A melting curve is introduced at the end of each amplification to exclude the presence of non specific binding between SYBER GREEN and primers.

2) *Immunohistochemistry.* Tissue sections need to be dewaxed and endogenous peroxidase activity blocked with 0.3% hydrogen peroxide in methanol for 15 min. For antigen retrieval, sections are immersed in 0.03 mol/L citrate buffer and incubated at 95 °C for 40 min. After rinsing in phosphate-buffered saline pH 7.2, 10% bovine serum is applied for 20 min to block non specific reactions. Sections are then incubated with a primary antibody (time and temperature of incubation depend on antibody characteristics). After rinsing in PBS, the sections are treated with peroxidase-labelled secondary antibody. The peroxidase reaction is visualized by incubating the sections with 0.02% 3,3'-diaminobenzidine tetrahydrochloride in 0.05 M Tris buffer with 0.01% hydrogen peroxide [23, 29, 30].

3) *In situ Hybridization (ISH)*. Generally, ISH is a type of hybridization that uses a labelled complementary DNA or RNA strand to localize a specific DNA or RNA sequence in a portion or section of tissue. This technique was used by Kammori *et al.* in 2003 [41] on formalin-fixed, paraffin-embedded tissue sections and FNAC samples, with a commercial kit (Genpoint nucleic acid hyperdetection system, Dako) and oligonuclotide probes synthesized with a hapten-labeled nucleotide (*i.e.* digoxigenin-dUTP) at 3' end. The probe sequence is: 5'-GCCTCGTCTTCTACAGGGAAGTTCACCACTGTCTT-3'

# miRNA

microRNA (miRNAs) are small (approximately 22 nucleotides), non-protein encoding RNAs that post-transcriptionally regulate gene expression *via* suppression of specific target mRNAs [44]. Recently, it was demonstrated that miRNAs circulate in a highly stable, cell-free form in blood and they can be measured in plasma and serum [45]. In addition, miRNAs can be released by tumour cells into the circulation [45] and profiles of miRNAs in plasma and serum have been found to be altered in cancer and other disease states [46-48]. Larger scale miRNAs analyses have shown that miRNA expression can differentiate benign tissues from their malignant counterparts [49, 50]. The mechanisms of miRNA implication in cancer development are linked to down-regulation of tumour suppressor genes or up-regulation of oncogenes (Fig. **3**).

Some studies have employed miRNA detection systems (microarray and/or Q-RT-PCR) to demonstrate unique molecular expression signatures of benign *versus* malignant thyroid lesions [51-54]. Tetzlaff *et al.* identified 13 up-regulated miRNAs and 26 down-regulated miRNAs in PTC *versus* multinodular goiter in formalin fixed paraffin-embedded tissues [51]. Among these, they found miRNA-21, miRNA-31, miRNA-221 and miRNA-222 [51]. Chen *et al.* [52] identified miRNA-146b,

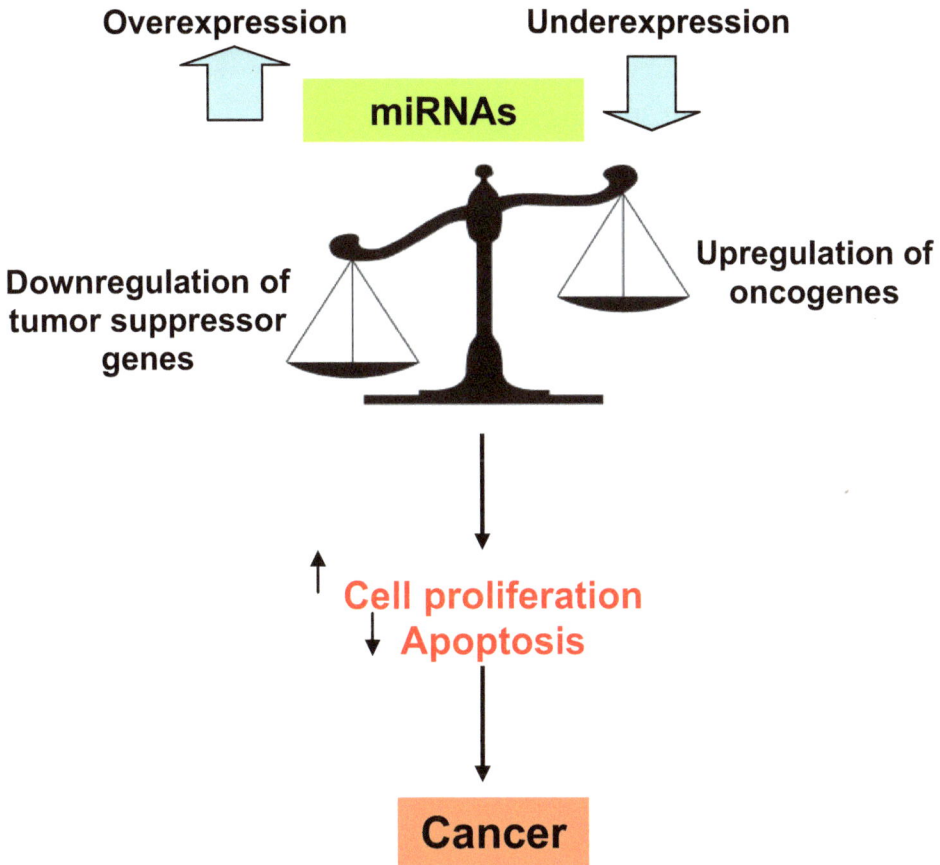

**Figure 3:** Role of miRNAs in cancer development.

miRNA-221 and miRNA-222 to be over expressed in PTC and found an increased expression of miRNA-146b in FTC both in fine-needle aspiration cytology (FNA) and surgical pathological specimens. The same mi-RNAs were found to be related to PTC formation in another study by He *et al.* [53]. In addition, in 2008, a set of seven miRNAs (miR-187, miR221, miR222, miR-146b, miR-155, miR-224 and miR-197) were found to be over-expressed in thyroid tumours compared to hyperplastic nodules both in the surgical and FNAC samples. Another article [55] demonstrated that a specific limited set of mi-RNAs (miRNA-197 and miRNA-346) is over-expressed in FTC in cell lines and tumour samples. Recently [56], different miRNAs have been explored in FNAC by Kitano *et al.* They evaluated miRNA7, miRNA126,

MiRNA374 and let7g. In this paper, miRNA7 was the best predictor to distinguish benign from malignant thyroid FNAC samples with a sensitivity of 100%, specificity of 29%, PPV of 36% and NPV of 100%.

All these studies concluded that a limited set of miRNAs can be used diagnostically for the differential diagnosis between benign and malignant lesions both in the surgical and pre-operative FNAC samples with high accuracy.

**Methods for the Analysis of miRNAs**

1.  *miRNA extraction and retro-transcription*: miRNAs are extracted from samples using specific commercial kits. Then, reverse transcription reactions are performed using TaqMan miRNA Reverse Transcription Kit and miRNA-specific stem loop primers (Applied Biosystem) in a 5 μl RT reaction [57]. Each tube contains 1.387 μl of water, 0.5 μl 10X Reverse-Transcription buffer, 0.063 μl RNase-Inhibitor (20 U/μl), 0.05 μl 100 mM dNTPs with dTTP, 0.33 μl Multiscribe Reverse Transcriptase, 1 μl RT primer. Tubes are mixed by inversion and briefly centrifuged. The RT reaction is carried out using the following conditions: 16°C for 30 minutes, 42 °C for 30 minutes, 85°C for 5 minutes and than hold at 4°C. RT products can be stored at -20°C until use.

2.  *Pre-amplification of RT products*: In some cases, to enhance sensitivity, the RT product can be pre-amplified prior to the real-time PCR step [58]. The pre-amplification step is carried out in a small-scale (5 μL) reaction comprised of 2.5 μl Taqman PreAmp Master Mix (2×), 1.25 μl Taqman miRNA assay (0.2×) (diluted in TE) and 1.25 μl undiluted RT product. For each miRNA-specific assay, a reaction pre-mix is prepared by combining sufficient Taqman PreAmp Master Mix (2X) and miRNA assay (0.2X) for all reactions. Samples are then mixed by inversion and centrifuged briefly. For each sample, 1.25 μl of the undiluted RT

product is added to the reaction pre-mix aliquots. Samples are mixed by inversion and centrifuged briefly. Pre-amplification is carried out on at these conditions: 95 °C for 10 min, followed by 14 cycles of 95 °C for 15 s and 60 °C for 4 min, followed by a hold at 4°C. The pre-amplification PCR product are diluted by adding 75 µl buffer TE1X and used in the Real Time amplification step [58].

3. *Real time PCR*: Real-time PCR reactions is performed in duplicate or triplicate, using 2.5 µl TaqMan 2× Universal PCR Master Mix, 0.25 µl miRNA-specific primer/probe mix, and 2.25 µl diluted RT product per reaction. Real-time PCR is carried out using the following conditions: 95°C for 10 min, followed by 40 cycles of 95°C for 15 s and 60°C for 1 min, followed by a hold at 4°C. It is possible generate a standard curve with synthetic miRNA. In this case, Ct values are plotted *versus* copy number of the synthetic miRNA in a standard curve allowing fitting of a curve that is used to approximate copies of endogenous miRNA from Ct values obtained with biological samples. In a different method, a miRNA generally expressed at same level in all tissues (*i.e.* miRNA U6) or rRNA 16S can be used to quantify miRNA of interest using the method of the $2^{-\Delta\Delta Ct}$. This method is defined as the quantification of expression levels obtained with a direct comparison of threshold cycles. The formula: $\Delta\Delta Ct$= Sample $\Delta Ct$-Reference $\Delta Ct$ can be explained as $\Delta Ct$ of Sample X analyzed for gene Y- $\Delta Ct$ of sample X analyzed for the reference gene [57, 59].

4. *Microarray expression analysis*: Generally, a microarray is a multiplex technology which consists of an arrayed series of thousands of microscopic spots of DNA oligonucleotides each containing picomoles of a specific DNA sequence. A gene sequence is used as probe to hybridize the cDNA of interest under high-stringency conditions. Probe-

target hybridization is detected and quantified by detection of fluorophore- or chemiluminescence-labeled targets to determine the presence/absence of the target. Specifically, biotin-labeled miRNA are hybridized on miRNA chips [60]. Briefly, 5 μg of total RNA from each sample are reverse transcribed by using biotin end-labeled octamers. Hybridization is carried out on microarray chips [53, 55] containing mature miRNA probes spotted at least in triplicate. Various preparations of the targets is described by Tetzlaff *et al.* [51]. After, chips are washed and processed to detect the labeled targets, scanned and quantified [51, 53, 55, 61-63].

## CONFLICT OF INTEREST

The author confirms that she has no conflicts of interest.

## ACKNOWLEDGEMENTS

Declared none.

## REFERENCES

[1]     Hundahl SA, Fleming ID, Fremgen AM, Menck HR. A National Cancer Data Base report on 53,856 cases of thyroid carcinoma treated in the U.S., 1985-1995. Cancer 1998, 83:2638-2648.

[2]     Begum S, Rosenbaum E, Henrique R, Cohen Y, Sidransky D, Westra WH. BRAF mutations in anaplastic thyroid carcinoma: implications for tumor origin, diagnosis and treatment. Mod Pathol 2004, 17:1359-63.

[3]     Cohen Y, Xing M, Mambo E, Guo Z, Wu G, Trink B, Beller U, Westra WH, Ladenson PW, Sidransky D. BRAF mutation in papillary thyroid carcinoma. J Natl Cancer Inst. 2003, 95:625-7.

[4]     Cheung L, Messina M, Gill A, Clarkson A, Learoyd D, Delbridge L, Wentworth J, Philips J, Clifton-Bligh R, Robinson BG. Detection of the PAX8-PPAR gamma fusion oncogene in both follicular thyroid carcinomas and adenomas. JCEM 2003, 88:354-7.

[5]     Dwight T, Thoppe SR, Foukakis T, Lui WO, Wallin G, Höög A, Frisk T, Larsson C, Zedenius J. Involvement of the PAX8/peroxisome proliferator-activated receptor gamma rearrangement in follicular thyroid tumors. JCEM 2003, 88:4440-5.

[6]   Esapa CT, Johnson SJ, Kendall-Taylor P, Lennard TW, Harris PE. Prevalence of Ras mutations in thyroid neoplasia. Clin Endocrinol (Oxf). 1999, 50:529-35.

[7]   Vasko V, Ferrand M, Di Cristofaro J, Carayon P, Henry JF, de Micco C. Specific pattern of RAS oncogene mutations in follicular thyroid tumors. JCEM 2003, 88:2745-52.

[8]   Zhu Z, Gandhi M, Nikiforova MN, Fischer AH, Nikiforov YE. Molecular profile and clinical-pathologic features of the follicular variant of papillary thyroid carcinoma. An unusually high prevalence of ras mutations. Am J Clin Pathol. 2003, 120:71-7.

[9]   Bounacer A, Wicker R, Caillou B, Cailleux AF, Sarasin A, Schlumberger M, Suárez HG. High prevalence of activating ret proto-oncogene rearrangements, in thyroid tumors from patients who had received external radiation. Oncogene 1997, 15:1263-73.

[10]  Elisei R, Romei C, Vorontsova T, Cosci B, Veremeychik V, Kuchinskaya E, Basolo F, Demidchik EP, Miccoli P, Pinchera A, Pacini F. RET/PTC rearrangements in thyroid nodules: studies in irradiated and not irradiated, malignant and benign thyroid lesions in children and adults. JCEM 2001, 86:3211-6.

[11]  Tallini G, Santoro M, Helie M, Carlomagno F, Salvatore G, Chiappetta G, Carcangiu ML, Fusco A. RET/PTC oncogene activation defines a subset of papillary thyroid carcinomas lacking evidence of progression to poorly differentiated or undifferentiated tumor phenotypes. Clin Cancer Res. 1998, 4:287-94.

[12]  Ju Z, Rudolph LK. Telomere dysfunction and stem cell ageing. Biochimie. 2008, 90:24-32.

[13]  Gilson E, Londono-Vallejo A. Telomere length profile in humans. Cell Cycle. 2007, 6:1–9.

[14]  Haugen BR, Nawaz S, Markham N, Hashizumi T, Shroyer AL, Werness B, Shroyer KR. Telomerase activity in benign and malignant thyroid tumors. Thyroid. 1997, 7:337–342.

[15]  Yashima K, Vuitch F, Gazdar AF, Fahey TJIII. Telomerase activity in benign and malignant thyroid diseases. Surgery. 1997, 122:1141–1146.

[16]  Kammori M, Takubo K, Nakamura KI, Furogouri E, Endo H, Kanauchi H, Mimura Y, Kaminishi M. Telomerase activity and telomere length in benign and malignant human thyroid tissues. Cancer Lett. 2000, 159:175–181.

[17]  Onoda N, Ishikawa T, Yoshikawa K, Sugano S, Kato Y, Sowa M, Hirakawa-Yong Suk Chung K. Telomerase activity in thyroid tumors. Oncol. Rep. 1998, 5:1447–1450.

[18]  Matthews P, Jones CJ, Skinner J, Haughton M, De Micco C, Wynford-Thomas D. Telomerase activity and telomere length in thyroid neoplasia: biological and clinical implications. J. Pathol. 2001, 194:183–193.

[19]  Aogi K, Kitahara K, Urquidi V, Tarin D, Goodison S. comparison of telomerase and CD44 expression as diagnostic tumor markers in lesions of the thyroid. Clin. Cancer Res. 1999, 5:2790–2797.

[20]  Lo CY, Lam KY, Chan KT, Luk JM. Telomerase activity in thyroid malignancy. Thyroid. 1999;9:1215–1220.

[21] Umbricht CB, Saji M, Westra WH, Udelsman R, Zeiger MA, Sukumar S. Telomerase activity: a marker to distinguish follicular thyroid adenoma from carcinoma. Cancer Res. 1997, 57:2144–2147.

[22] Brousset P, Chaouche N, Leprat F, Branet-Brousset F, Trouette H, Zenou RC, Merlio JP, Delsol G. Telomerase activity in human thyroid carcinomas originating from the follicular cells. J. Clin. Endocrinol. Metab. 1997, 82:4214–4216.

[23] Hoang-Vu C, Boltze C, Gimm O, Poremba C, Dockhorn-dworniczak B, Kohrle J, Rath FW, Dralle H. Expression of telomerase genes in thyroid carcinoma. Int. J. Oncol. 2002, 21:265–272.

[24] Saji M, Xydas S, Westra WH, Liang CK, Clark DP, Udelsman R, Umbricht CB, Sukumar S, Zeiger MA. Human telomerase reverse transcriptase (hTERT) gene expression in thyroid neoplasms. Clin. Cancer Res. 1999, 5:1483–1489.

[25] Okayasu I, Osakabe T, Fujiwara M, Fukuda H, Kato M, Oshimura M. Significant correlation of telomerase activity in thyroid papillary carcinomas with cell differentiation, proliferation and extrathyroidal extension. Jpn. J. Cancer Res. 1997, 88:965–70.

[26] Bornstein-Quevedo L, Garcia-Hernandez ML, Camacho-Arroyo I, Herrera MF, Angeles AA, Trevino OG, Gam-boa-Dominguez A. Telomerase activity in well-differentiated papillary thyroid carcinoma correlates with advanced clinical stage of the disease. Endocr. Pathol. 2003, 14:213–219.

[27] Cheng AJ, Lin JD, Chang T, Wang TCV. Telomerase activity in benign and malignant human thyroid tissues. Br. J. Cancer. 1998, 77:2177–2180.

[28] Zeiger MA, Smallridge RC, Clark DP, Liang CK, Carty SE, Watson CG, Udelsman R, Saji M. Human telomerase reverse transcriptase (hTERT) gene expression in FNA samples from thyroid neoplasms. Surgery. 1999, 126:1195–1199.

[29] Ito Y, Yoshida H, Tomoda C, Uruno T, Takamura Y, Miya A, Kobayashi K, Matsuzuka F, Kuma K, Miyauchi A. Telomerase activity in thyroid neoplasms evaluated by the expression of human telomerase reverse transcriptase (hTERT) Anticancer Res. 2005, 25:509–514.

[30] Wang SL, Chen WT, Wu MT, Chan HM, Yang SF, Chai CY. Expression of human telomerase reverse transcriptase in thyroid follicular neoplasms: an immunohistochemical study. Endocr. Pathol. 2005, 16:211–218.

[31] Takano T, Ito Y, Matsuzuka F, Miya A, Kobayashi K, Yoshida H, Miyauchi A. Quantitative measurement of telomerase reverse transcriptase, thyroglobulin and thyroid transcription factor 1 mRNAs in anaplastic thyroid carcinoma tissues and cell lines. Oncol. Rep. 2007, 18:715–720.

[32] Mitomo S, Maesawa C, Ogasawara S, Iwaya T, Shibazaki M, Yashima-Abo A, Kotani K, Oikawa H, Sakurai E, Izutsu N, Kato K, Komatsu H, Ikeda K, Wakabayashi G, Masuda T. Downregulation of miR-138 is associated with overexpression of human telomerase reverse

transcriptase protein in human anaplastic thyroid carcinoma cell lines. Cancer Sci. 2008, 99:280–6.

[33]   Straight AM, Patel A, Fenton C, Dinauer C, Tuttle RM, Francis GL. Thyroid carcinomas that express telomerase follow a more aggressive clinical course in children and adolescents. J. Endorinol. Invest. 2002, 25:302–308.

[34]   Foukakis T, Gusnanto A, Au AY, Hoog A, Lui WO, Larsson C, Wallin G, Zedenius J. A PCR-based expression signature of malignancy in follicular thyroid tumors. Endocr. Relat. Cancer. 2007, 14:381–391.

[35]   Aogi K, Kitahara K, Buley I, Backdahal M, Tahara H, Sugino T, Tarin D, Goodison S. Telomerase activity in lesions of the thyroid: application to diagnosis of clinical samples including fine-needle aspirates. Clin. Cancer Res. 1998, 4:1965–1970.

[36]   Sebesta J, Brown T, Williard W, Dehart MJ, Aldous W, Kavolius J, Azarow K. Does telomerase add to the value of fine needle aspirations in evaluating thyroid nodules? Am. J. Surg. 2001, 181:420–422.

[37]   Mora J, Lerma E. Thyroid Neoplasia Study Group. Telomerase activity in thyroid fine needle apirates. Acta Cytol. 2004, 48:818–824.

[38]   Lerma E, Mora J. Telomerase activity in "suspicious" thyroid cytology. Cancer. 2005, 10:492–497.

[39]   Trulsson LM, Velin AK, Herder A, Söderkvist P, Rüter A, Smeds S. Telomerase activity in surgical specimens and fine-needle aspiration biopsies from hyperplastic and neoplastic human thyroid tissues. Am. J. Surg. 2003, 186:83–8.

[40]   Guerra LN, Miler EA, Moiguer S, Karner M, Orlandi AM, Fideleff H, Burdman JA. Telomerase activity in fine needle aspiration biopsy samples: application to diagnosis of human thyroid carcinoma. Clin. Chim. Acta. 2006, 370:180–184.

[41]   Kammori M, Nakamura K, Hashimoto M, Ogawa T, Kaminishi M, Takubo K. Clinical application of human telomerase reverse transcriptase gene expression in thyroid follicular tumors by fine-needle aspirations using *in situ* hybridization. Int J Oncol. 2003, 22:985–991.

[42]   Capezzone M, Cantara S, Marchisotta S, Filetti S, De Santi MM, Rossi B, Ronga G, Durante C, Pacini F. Short telomeres, telomerase reverse transcriptase gene amplification, and increased telomerase activity in the blood of familial papillary thyroid cancer patients. JCEM 2008, 93:3950-7.

[43]   Kim NW, Piatyszek MA, Prowse KR, Harley CB, West MD, Ho PL, Coviello GM, Wright WE, Weinrich SL, Shay JW. Specific association of human telomerase activity with immortal cells and cancer. Science 1994, 266:2011-5.

[44]   Carthew RW, Sontheimer EJ. Origins and Mechanisms of miRNAs and siRNAs. Cell 2009, 136:642-655.

[45]   Mitchell PS, Parkin RK, Kroh EM, Fritz BR, Wyman SK, Pogosova-Agadjanyan EL, Peterson A, Noteboom J, O'Briant KC, Allen A, Lin DW, Urban N, Drescher CW, Knudsen

BS, Stirewalt DL, Gentleman R, Vessella RL, Nelson PS, Martin DB, Tewari M. Circulating microRNAs as stable blood-based markers for cancer detection. PNAS 2008, 105:10513-10518.

[46]    Chen X, Ba Y, Ma L, Cai X, Yin Y, Wang K, Guo J, Zhang Y, Chen J, Guo X, Li Q, Li X, Wang W, Zhang Y, Wang J, Jiang X, Xiang Y, Xu C, Zheng P, Zhang J, Li R, Zhang H, Shang X, Gong T, Ning G, Wang J, Zen K, Zhang J, Zhang CY. Characterization of microRNAs in serum: a novel class of biomarkers for diagnosis of cancer and other diseases. Cell Res. 2008, 18:997-1006.

[47]    Lawrie CH, Gal S, Dunlop HM, Pushkaran B, Liggins AP, Pulford K, Banham AH, Pezzella F, Boultwood J, Wainscoat JS, Hatton CS, Harris AL. Detection of elevated levels of tumour-associated microRNAs in serum of patients with diffuse large B-cell lymphoma. Br J Haematol. 2008, 141:672-5.

[48]    Taylor DD, Gercel-Taylor C. MicroRNA signatures of tumor-derived exosomes as diagnostic biomarkers of ovarian cancer. Gynecol Oncol. 2008, 110:13-21.

[49]    Lu J, Getz G, Miska EA, Alvarez-Saavedra E, Lamb J, Peck D, Sweet-Cordero A, Ebert BL, Mak RH, Ferrando AA, Downing JR, Jacks T, Horvitz HR, Golub TR. MicroRNA expression profiles classify human cancers. Nature 2005, 435:834-8.

[50]    Volinia S, Calin GA, Liu CG, Ambs S, Cimmino A, Petrocca F, Visone R, Iorio M, Roldo C, Ferracin M, Prueitt RL, Yanaihara N, Lanza G, Scarpa A, Vecchione A, Negrini M, Harris CC, Croce CM. A microRNA expression signature of human solid tumors defines cancer gene targets. PNAS 2006, 103:2257-61.

[51]    Tetzlaff MT, Liu A, Xu X, Master SR, Baldwin DA, Tobias JW, Livolsi VA, Baloch ZW. Differential expression of miRNAs in papillary thyroid carcinoma compared to multinodular goiter using formalin fixed paraffin embedded tissues. Endocr Pathol 2007, 18:163-173.

[52]    Chen YT, Kitabayashi N, Zhou XK, Fahey TJ 3rd, Scognamiglio T. MicroRNA analysis as a potential diagnostic tool for papillary thyroid carcinoma. Mod Pathol. 2008, 21:1139-1146.

[53]    He H, Jazdzewski K, Li W, Liyanarachchi S, Nagy R, Volinia S, Calin GA, Liu CG, Franssila K, Suster S, Kloos RT, Croce CM, de la Chapelle A. The role of microRNA genes in papillary thyroid carcinoma. PNAS 2005, 102:19075-19080.

[54]    Nikifororva MN, Tseng GC, Steward D, Diorio D, Nikiforov Y. MicroRNA expression profiling of thyroid tumors: biological significance and diagnostic utility. JCEM 2008, 93:1600-8.

[55]    Weber F, Teresi RE, Broelsch CE, Frilling A, Eng C. A limited set of human MicroRNA is deregulated in follicular thyroid carcinoma. JCEM 2006, 91:3584-91.

[56]    Kitano M, Rahbari R, Patterson EE, Steinberg SM, Prasad NB, Wang Y, Zeiger MA, Kebebew E. Evaluation of Candidate diagnostic microRNAs in thyroid fine-needle aspiration biopsy samples. Thyroid 2012, 22:285-91.

[57]    Chen C, Ridzon DA, Broomer AJ, Zhou Z, Lee DH, Nguyen JT, Barbisin M, Xu NL, Mahuvakar VR, Andersen MR, Lao KQ, Livak KJ, Guegler KJ. Real-time quantification of microRNAs by stem-loop RT-PCR. Nucleic Acids Res. 2005, 33:e179.

[58]    Kroh EM, Parkin RK, Mitchell PS, Tewari M. Analysis of circulating microRNA biomarkers in plasma and serum using quantitative reverse transcription-PCR (qRT-PCR). Methods 2010, 50:298-301.

[59]    Raymond CK, Roberts BS, Garrett-Engele P, Lim LP, Johnson JM. Simple, quantitative primer-extension PCR assay for direct monitoring of microRNAs and short-interfering RNAs. RNA. 2005, 11:1737-44.

[60]    Liu CG, Calin GA, Meloon B, Gamliel N, Sevignani C, Ferracin M, Dumitru CD, Shimizu M, Zupo S, Dono M, Alder H, Bullrich F, Negrini M, Croce CM. An oligonucleotide microchip for genome-wide microRNA profiling in human and mouse tissues. PNAS 2004, 101:9740-9744.

[61]    Weber F, Shen L, Aldred MA, Morrison CD, Frilling A, Saji M, Schuppert F, Broelsch CE, Ringel MD, Eng C. Genetic classification of benign and malignant thyroid follicular neoplasia based on a three-gene combination. JCEM 2005, 90:2512-2521.

[62]    Aldred MA, Huang Y, Liyanarachchi S, Pellegata NS, Gimm O, Jhiang S, Davuluri RV, de la Chapelle A, Eng C. Papillary and follicular thyroid carcinomas show distinctly different microarray expression profiles and can be distinguished by a minimum of five genes. J Clin Oncol 2004, 22:3531-3539.

[63]    Auer H, Lyianarachchi S, Newsom D, Klisovic MI, Marcucci G, Kornacker K. Chipping away at the chip bias: RNA degradation in microarray analysis. Nat Genet 2003, 35:292-293.

# APPENDIX

After writing the eBook, I must point out that, especially with regard to the chapters inherent the molecular biology procedures, I cannot exclude that these may change in future and some of the techniques described may become old and obsolete. Anyway, the described PCR primers, cycles and the given tool and indications will last and could be of great help just for the validation of new future methodologies.

# Subject Index

**A**

Axitinib 90

**B**

BRAF oncogene 30-32, 49-53, 57-58, 77

**C**

Cabozantinib 90-91

Calcitonin 5, 6-7, 9, 77

Carney Complex 66

CD44v6 18

Ck-19 18

Cowden disease 66

**E**

Elastography 8

**F**

FAP 65-66

Fine needle aspiration 5, 8, 15

Familial medullary thyroid cancer 78-79

Familial non medullary thyroid cancer 64-71

**G**

Galectin-3 16-17

**H**

HBME-1 17-18